Death, Dying, and Organ Transplantation

Death, Dying, and Organ Transplantation

*Reconstructing Medical Ethics
at the End of Life*

FRANKLIN G. MILLER

AND

ROBERT D. TRUOG

OXFORD
UNIVERSITY PRESS

OXFORD
UNIVERSITY PRESS

Oxford University Press, Inc., publishes works that further
Oxford University's objective of excellence
in research, scholarship, and education.

Oxford New York
Auckland   Cape Town   Dar es Salaam   Hong Kong   Karachi
Kuala Lumpur   Madrid   Melbourne   Mexico City   Nairobi
New Delhi   Shanghai   Taipei   Toronto

With offices in
Argentina   Austria   Brazil   Chile   Czech Republic   France   Greece
Guatemala   Hungary   Italy   Japan   Poland   Portugal   Singapore
South Korea   Switzerland   Thailand   Turkey   Ukraine   Vietnam

Copyright © 2012 Oxford University Press

Published by Oxford University Press, Inc.
198 Madison Avenue, New York, New York 10016

www.oup.com

Oxford is a registered trademark of Oxford University Press

Library of Congress Cataloging-in-Publication Data

Miller, Franklin G.
Death, dying, and organ transplantation : reconstructing medical ethics
at the end of life / Franklin G. Miller and Robert D. Truog.
    p. ; cm.
ISBN 978-0-19-973917-2
1. Euthanasia—Moral and ethical aspects. 2. Procurement of organs,
tissues, etc.—Moral and ethical aspects. I. Truog, Robert. II. Title.
[DNLM: 1. Withholding Treatment—ethics. 2. Ethics, Medical.
3. Euthanasia, Active—ethics. 4. Tissue and Organ Procurement—ethics. WB 60]
R726.M5525 2011
179.7—dc22   2011003572

CONTENTS

Modern medicine has achieved an exalted status in contemporary society, in large part because of its technological prowess in preserving life. Two of the most notable examples are the interventions performed in intensive care units (ICUs) and organ transplantation. While the life-preserving powers of medicine reflected in these two examples have been lauded, it has not been widely recognized that these powers go hand in hand with practices that (legitimately) cause the death of patients: withdrawing life-sustaining treatment, such as ventilators, dialysis, and feeding tubes, and procuring vital organs for transplantation. The death-causing flip-side, so to speak, of these forms of life-preserving technology has been obscured by fundamental commitments of established medical ethics at the end of life: the traditional norm that clinicians must not kill their patients and "the dead donor rule," which prescribes that vital organs can be procured only from dead human beings. A semblance of coherence between the practices of withdrawing life support and procuring vital organs and established medical ethics has been maintained by understanding treatment withdrawal as merely allowing patients to die and by transforming the traditional medical criteria for determining death, such that vital organ donors are declared dead prior to organ procurement.

In this book we argue that the conventional accounts of withdrawing life-sustaining treatment and procuring vital organs are mistaken: both involve causing the death of patients. Our aim is not to challenge the ethical legitimacy of these practices but to demonstrate that medical ethics needs to be reconstructed so that it harmonizes with the reality of these practices. In facing up to the reality of common medical practices at the end of life we are not left with an ethical vacuum. Ethical resources are readily available to justify causing death by withdrawing life support and procuring vital organs from still living patients. To do so, however, requires abandoning the absolute norm that clinicians must not intentionally cause the death of their patients and the dead donor rule.

Often moral progress comes from giving up practices that conflict with established or evolving moral norms, as in the movements for civil rights for historically disadvantaged minority groups and gender equality. In other cases, moral progress can come from recognizing that established norms are unsuitable because they are incompatible with the reality of ethically legitimate common practices. Established norms are not always justified, or may need to be revised or reconstructed. When legitimate institutional practices deviate from faulty norms, what is needed is to change the norms, not to abandon norm-conflicting practices. Such is the situation we face with respect to medical ethics at the end of life.

PLAN AND OUTLINE OF THE BOOK

In Chapter 1 we discuss withdrawing life-sustaining treatment. The argument that this routine practice causes the death of patients, rather than merely allows them to die from their underlying medical condition, sets the stage for the ethical analysis that we deploy throughout the book. We contend that the patent causal contribution of treatment withdrawal to the timing of patients' deaths and the intentions of clinicians involved in this practice are obscured by a morally biased description of the facts, which is driven by the continued commitment to the traditional norm of medical ethics that doctors must not intentionally cause the death of their patients.

We take up the ethics of active euthanasia in Chapter 2. Appreciation that withdrawing life support causes the death of patients undermines the traditional bright lines in medical ethics that distinguish this legitimate practice and palliative care from the allegedly illegitimate practice of active euthanasia by lethal injection. Considerable attention is devoted to assessing active euthanasia in light of an account of the role morality and the professional integrity of physicians, which have to a large extent been neglected in philosophical treatments of this issue. We argue that professional integrity does not preclude active euthanasia but limits this practice to interventions of last resort for relieving the suffering of incurably ill patients. Policy considerations relating to legalization of active euthanasia are addressed as well.

In Chapters 3 and 4 we undertake an extended analysis of the determination of death on the basis of neurological criteria, which plays a central role in the prevailing justification for transplantation of vital organs. Drawing on knowledge regarding the functioning of individuals who meet the diagnostic criteria for "brain death," we contend that they are not dead in accordance with the established biological conception of death in terms of the cessation of the integrative functioning of the organism as a whole. A recent attempt by a U.S.

bioethics commission to uphold the neurological criteria for determining death by developing a novel account of why "brain dead" individuals are dead fails to withstand critical scrutiny. In Chapter 4 we defend the traditional basis for determining death by means of circulatory and respiratory criteria from objections that it leads to the allegedly absurd conclusion that decapitated human bodies may remain alive. In the second half of this chapter we discuss critically the "higher brain" standard of death, espoused by some philosophers and bioethicists, which makes loss of the capacity for consciousness the key to the death of human beings.

Chapter 5 is devoted to a critical account of the application of circulatory and respiratory criteria for determining death to vital organ donation following withdrawal of life-sustaining treatment—a growing practice driven by the inadequate supply of organs from "brain dead" donors. This approach to determining death, only a very short interval after the donor's heart has stopped beating, founders by fudging the requirement that cessation of circulatory functioning must be irreversible. Efforts to establish the credibility for determination of death in this context are found unconvincing.

Although the dead donor rule has been adopted as an ethical axiom, the upshot of Chapters 3 and 5 is that "brain dead" donors remain alive and donors declared dead according to circulatory–respiratory criteria are not known to be dead at the time that their organs are procured. Either vital organ donation must cease because it is seen as unethical, which would be a drastic outcome, or an ethical justification is needed that does not rely on the dead donor rule. The critique of prevailing justificatory accounts for current end-of-life practices in preceding chapters paves the way for constructive approaches to justifying vital organ donation in Chapters 6 and 7. In Chapter 6 we develop an account of the ethics of vital organ donation from still-living donors contingent on valid plans to withdraw life-sustaining treatment and consent. Under these circumstances, donors are not harmed or wronged by organ procurement prior to stopping treatment. We defend this ethical approach by taking up a series of challenging objections. In Chapter 7, written with Seema Shah, J.D. (and based on Shah and Miller 2010), we develop a pragmatic alternative justificatory account based on the concept of legal fictions. We analyze current practices of vital organ donation as based on unacknowledged legal fictions that underlie determinations of death prior to organ procurement. As a way of approaching the ideal goal of honest engagement with the legitimacy of vital organ donation from still-living patients, we advocate making these legal fictions transparent by acknowledging that death in the eyes of the law is not the same as death in fact according to a biological definition.

We close the book with an epilogue, which briefly sums up the project of reconstructing medical ethics at the end of life.

ACKNOWLEDGMENTS

Much of the territory covered in this book was initially mapped in several previously published collaborative papers (Miller and Truog 2008; 2009; 2010; Miller et al. 2010a, 2010b; and Shah and Miller 2010). We appreciate the astute intellectual contributions of Dan Brock, co-author of two of these papers. The discussion of professional integrity, which plays a prominent role in Chapters Two and Six, draws heavily on some of Miller's previous collaborations with Howard Brody (Miller and Brody 1995; 2001). We thank Bob Goodin and Jim Nelson for thoughtful comments on previous drafts of Chapter Six. Finally, Miller dedicates his work on this book to the memory of his sister Debbie, whose courageous life in the face of quadriplegia and planned death inspired reflections on withdrawing life-sustaining treatment, causing death, and organ donation.

Withdrawing Life-Sustaining Treatment

Allowing to Die or Causing Death?

The advent of the mechanical ventilator in the mid-twentieth century and the institutional setting of the intensive care unit forced clinicians, ethicists, and the law to face the unprecedented problem of whether, and under what conditions, it is legitimate to withdraw life-sustaining medical treatment (LST). Since at least the time of the Quinlan case in 1976, withdrawing life-sustaining treatment has been publicly considered a legally and ethically legitimate practice, which respects the rights of patients to self-determination. Competent patients are entitled to refuse or to withdraw consent for any medical treatment. When they become incapable of deciding for themselves, this right is exercised by surrogate decision makers, typically family members, with the decision to continue or cease LST based on the preferences and values of the patient, if known, or what is deemed to be in the patient's best interest. Along with endorsing this ethical stance, grounded in patient self-determination and personal well-being, medicine, medical ethics, and the law have continued to embrace the traditional norm that doctors must never intentionally kill their patients. Accordingly, withdrawing LST has been widely regarded as allowing the patient to die and *not* as causing death. We contend that this stance cannot withstand critical scrutiny because withdrawing life-sustaining treatment, when examined without moral preconceptions, is clearly seen as causing death. Although our critique of the conventional understanding of withdrawing LST as merely allowing the patient to die does not call into question the ethical justification of this practice in terms of patient self-determination and personal well-being, it has an important implication for medical ethics: medicine should no longer be governed by the norm that doctors must not intentionally cause the death of their patients. In other words, medical ethics should be reconstructed so that it can accommodate the routine practice of withdrawing LST understood as legitimately causing death.

For some readers, our extended argument in this chapter for the proposition that withdrawing LST causes death may seem to demonstrate merely what is obvious. Yet the view that withdrawing LST merely allows patients to die and does not cause death is deeply entrenched in conventional medical ethics. Moreover, it is a central thesis of this book that understanding the common practice of withdrawing LST as causing death has important ethical implications for thinking about active euthanasia and organ donation. Hence, establishing that withdrawal of life support causes death is pivotal to the position that we advance.

Independent of conventional medical ethics, there is an extensive philosophical literature on killing and letting die, encompassing a variety of subtle and complex conceptual analyses and arguments (Steinbock and Norcross 1994; Kamm 1996; McMahan 2002). We do not discuss this literature in depth, as our focus is on standard views in conventional medical ethics.

CAUSING DEATH

The traditional norm in medicine relating to causing death is typically described as "Doctors must not kill" (Gaylin et al. 1988). There are two ways in which medical conduct associated with the death of patients can escape the scope of this norm. First, it can be denied that the conduct in question causes death. Second, it can be denied that death is caused intentionally. We will examine critically the prevailing view of withdrawing LST in medical ethics in terms of both these ways of characterizing this practice.

At first glance, withdrawing LST may not appear to cause death because it differs from paradigmatic cases of killing. Typical killings involve an agent B producing a physical impact on A that, by itself, is sufficient to cause A's death. B kills A by stabbing, strangling, shooting with a gun, poisoning, lethal injection, etc. In other words, the agent directly *induces* the victim's death by some physical intervention. In withdrawing LST, such as a mechanical ventilator, a clinician sets in motion a causal chain leading to the patient's death by virtue of the fact that the patient has a disease or injury that makes it impossible to live in the absence of LST. (We will explain below how withdrawing artificial nutrition and hydration has a somewhat different causal connection with death.) Although death is not directly induced by withdrawing LST, it doesn't follow that the act of stopping treatment merely allows the patient to die and does not cause, or contribute to causing, the patient's death.

In general, we will be arguing that withdrawing LST "causes death" rather than "kills," owing to the way that "killing" is used in the medical context. In this context, "killing" is commonly understood as meaning the *wrongful* taking of life (President's Commission 1983, 64), despite the fact that nearly everyone recognizes that killing can be justified in other contexts, such as self-defense and a just war. In view of this connotation in the medical context, it seems jarring to describe withdrawing life support as killing, and it interferes with an impartial appraisal of causing death. There is another related reason for not describing withdrawing LST as killing. In paradigm cases of killing, both unjustified and justified, A *takes* B's life when A kills B. We argue that the clinician who withdraws LST, in accordance with the valid consent of the patient or a surrogate deciding on an incompetent patient's behalf, causes the patient's death. But surely in this situation the clinician does not take the patient's life in the sense of intervening without authorization. Likewise, voluntary active euthanasia is agreed by all to cause death but also does not take the patient's life, as the responsible clinician responds to the patient's request for help in dying and consent to a life-terminating intervention. Other cases of justified killing, such as self-defense, just war, and (possibly) capital punishment, do involve taking life. The killing, though justified, is not authorized by the one who is killed. Although it is certainly possible to distinguish between authorized and unauthorized killings, the usual connotations of "killing" suggest taking life without authorization. "Causing death" is more naturally used in a normatively neutral sense, with no implications relating to justification or authorization.

People investigate and assign causes in the process of explaining events. Causation is investigated and assigned for a variety of purposes: curiosity, to understand why and how an untoward event occurred in order to prevent such events from happening in the future, to determine liability for wrongdoing, etc. We suggest that the major reason why withdrawing LST is not seen as causing death according to the prevailing view in medical ethics is that causation in this context is typically approached with respect to the issue of liability for wrongdoing. Clinicians do no wrong in withdrawing LST when competent and informed patients refuse treatment or when authorized surrogates legitimately refuse it on their behalf. Indeed, they are obligated to withdraw treatment in order to respect the rights of patients. Because they do no wrong, and causing death is generally considered to be wrongful, it is assumed that they have not caused death. But this confuses and conflates causation and culpability. We attribute this mistake to what we call *moral bias*, explained below, in which commitment to the norm that clinicians must not kill their patients produces the skewed belief that clinicians are not causing death when they legitimately withdraw LST.

Withdrawing LST, such as a ventilator or dialysis, is a causal factor that, along with the patient's underlying medical condition, explains the occurrence of a patient's death at a given time. For without the withdrawal, the patient would have continued to live for either a short or prolonged period of time. Thus, it is misleading to characterize withdrawing LST as only allowing the patient to die and not as causing death. Both actively causing death and passively allowing a patient to die involve what Foot called "a fatal sequence"—a trajectory of events that ends in someone's death (Foot 1994, 283). What distinguishes the former from the latter is that in actively causing death the agent initiates the fatal sequence, as distinct from merely permitting it to continue without intervention to stop it.

Consider the situation of a 30-year-old ventilator-dependent patient with high-level spinal cord injury who has been admitted to the hospital to treat sepsis resulting from an infection. Suppose that this patient, after his sepsis has cleared and before discharge from the hospital, judges on the basis of careful deliberation that continued living with profound disability and burdensome life support is no longer worthwhile and therefore decides to stop treatment. Assuming that the patient is competent, clinicians not only may respect his decision but are obliged to respect his decision to withdraw LST. Fifteen minutes after the ventilator is stopped, the patient dies. We argue that withdrawing LST in this case patently causes the patient's death because it initiates the fatal sequence leading to death at the time it occurs, and that it is a mistake to claim that it merely allows the patient to die. Absent the withdrawal, the patient likely would continue to live for an extended period of time, perhaps decades. The clinician who turns off the ventilator does not merely stand by and permit the patient's spinal cord injury to cause death. To be sure, once the ventilator is stopped, then clinicians stand by, thus allowing the patient to die. But, to repeat, the treatment withdrawal initiates this fatal sequence.

Our focus on withdrawing LST in cases of ventilator-dependent patients with quadriplegia might be criticized as not representative of most medical situations in which LST is withdrawn. This is true, as these patients have a prognosis of living for a substantial period of time with continued mechanical ventilation, whereas in the typical case in which life support is withdrawn in the medical intensive care unit, patients have a poor prognosis and are likely to die in a short period of time despite aggressive treatment (Zussman 1992, 123–138). However, several of the most important "right to die" cases have involved patients in a permanent vegetative state, such as Karen Quinlan and Nancy Cruzan, who can live for a long time with artificial feeding and hydration and good nursing care (Pence 1995). The prevailing view that withdrawing LST does not cause death has been propounded as a universal proposition applying to all cases when physicians have no duty to continue treatment.

With respect to patients who could live indefinitely with continued LST, it is most patent that withdrawing LST causes death. Recognizing that it causes death in the case of these patients points the way to seeing that it also does so, at least as a contributory cause, in more typical cases, where death is hastened (made to occur sooner than it otherwise would) by the withdrawal of treatment.

Brock proposed the following thought experiment to demonstrate that withdrawing the ventilator causes the patient's death (Brock 1993, 209–210). Suppose that a person plotting the death of the patient with quadriplegia described above entered the patient's room and "pulled the plug." He would be guilty of murder—of wrongfully causing the death of the patient. It would obviously be disingenuous for him to say that he merely allowed the patient to die. Although there is all the difference in the world, morally speaking, between the act of murder by the patient's enemy and the valid treatment withdrawal by a clinician, it is difficult to see how in the former case the patient's death is caused by the perpetrator pulling the plug but is not caused by the same act performed by a doctor.

Another way to see that withdrawing LST causes death is to reflect on the concept of effective life-sustaining treatment. A medical intervention works to produce a given clinical outcome by means of a causal process. For example, mechanical ventilation saves or sustains the lives of patients with respiratory failure by an intervention that causes the body to continue breathing when otherwise respiration and circulation would cease and death would ensue. It follows that when mechanical ventilation is stopped, a patient who is incapable of breathing spontaneously will die. Stopping the ventilator contributes causally to the occurrence of death. To be sure, as discussed in some detail below, stopping LST, such as a ventilator, typically results in death only for patients who have an underlying medical condition for which treatment is needed to sustain life. But it does not follow that it is this condition alone that causes death when the ventilator is stopped. For if life support were continued, the patient likely would continue to live (in some cases for a prolonged period of time).

It may be objected that since LST operates to arrest a natural process of dying from disease or injury that would otherwise proceed to death, stopping the ventilator merely allows the natural dying process to proceed. But if implementing LST, such as a ventilator, can arrest the natural process of dying—it causes that process to cease or slows its progression—then when it is stopped, the withdrawal sets in motion a new causal process (a fatal sequence) that leads to death. Removing a barrier to a causal process is itself a cause of the outcome that ensues after the barrier is removed, especially when the barrier has the ability to arrest the process for a considerable period of time. Whereas withholding mechanical ventilation from a patient who has refused it merely allows the patient to die, this is not true of the act of turning off the ventilator that has been sustaining life for a patient who now refuses to continue this treatment. The former is an omission of treatment; the latter is a deliberate intervention to stop treatment. Withholding and withdrawing LST are considered to be *morally* equivalent—a judgment with which we concur; nevertheless, withdrawing LST is not the same from a *causal* perspective as standing by while the natural process of dying proceeds unchecked to death, as in withholding treatment.

In other situations we readily explain the cause of an outcome in reference to the stopping of a mechanical intervention. Consider the following example. A sailboat springs a leak and begins to take on water. The sailor turns on a battery-operated pump that keeps the boat from filling up with water. The battery, however, becomes drained and the pump stops working. The boat begins to fill up with water. What caused this outcome? Obviously, it wouldn't have happened if the boat hadn't sprung a leak. But it also wouldn't have happened if the pump had continued to operate. Thus, it is natural to say that the stopping of the pump (along with the leak) caused the boat to fill up with water. At the least, we would note the battery failure as contributing causally to, or being a partial cause of, the outcome. If the stopping of the pump by battery failure causes the boat to fill up with water, then certainly the same outcome would be caused if the sailor, for some reason, turned off the pump. Once a mechanical device intervenes to arrest a natural process, the stopping of the device causally explains, at least in part, the outcome. If not *the* cause, it is a cause. It is difficult to see why the same account should not apply to stopping LST, such as mechanical ventilation.

In arguing that withdrawing LST causes a patient's death, we do not adopt any particular philosophical or scientific theory of causation; rather, we appeal to our common-sense understanding of the causes of particular events, which has been astutely analyzed by Hart and Honore (1985) in their classic text, *Causation in the Law*. They note that "The notion, that a cause is essentially something which interferes with or intervenes in the course of events which would normally take place, is central to the common-sense concept of cause" (29). Causes are events or circumstances that *make the difference* in explaining a particular occurrence. Assuming that when a patient is on life support, the patient normally will continue to live for some period of time (though may be vulnerable to dying despite LST), then withdrawing life support is an intervention that brings about death, when death, in fact, ensues after the withdrawal occurs. The withdrawal makes the difference between continued living and death occurring at a given time subsequent to the withdrawal. In discussing inquiries relating to the cause of death, Hart and Honore observe that what is wanted is to "explain *this* man's death *now*" (40). Accordingly, the underlying medical condition (e.g., the incapacity for spontaneous breathing) is not eligible as *the* cause of the patient's death, as it operates both while the patient is on life support and after support is withdrawn.

Consider two patients in an intensive care unit with the same medical condition both of whom need mechanical ventilation to survive. For patient A, a family member decides to stop treatment, appealing to the patient's expressed preferences. For patient B, a family member insists on continued treatment as consistent with this patient's preferences. A dies 1 hour after the ventilator is turned off; B continues to live. We contend that it is incoherent to hold that it is not the withdrawal of LST but the underlying medical condition that causes the death of A, as B with the very same medical condition continues to live. Once again, the treatment withdrawal makes the difference. A fatal sequence has been initiated for patient A; patient B continues to live.

It is all the more difficult to maintain that withdrawing LST does not cause the death of patients when artificial nutrition and hydration is the treatment that is withdrawn, as in the case of Nancy Cruzan. In these situations, it is more of a stretch to appeal to the underlying medical condition as the cause of death; rather, the patient dies as a result of dehydration, subsequent to the withdrawal of artificial nutrition and hydration. The underlying medical condition helps to explain why the patient is not able to eat or drink on her own, but not why the patient becomes dehydrated. The death results from the withdrawal of LST and subsequent dehydration. It is for this reason that some commentators who view withdrawal of other forms of LST as allowing patients to die but not causing their death take a different position on withdrawing artificial nutrition and hydration, seeing it as causing the patient's death (Brody 1996).

Reviewing the history of medical thinking with respect to withdrawing LST bolsters the rationale for rejecting the factual claim in the prevailing view of medical ethics that withdrawing LST does not cause death. There is evidence that at least prior to the Quinlan case in 1976, doctors commonly regarded stopping LST such as mechanical ventilation as causing death (or at least feared that it would be so regarded) and thus would make them liable for criminal homicide. We suggest that these concerns about withdrawing treatment were reasonable precisely because the practice does cause death, though this fact is perfectly consistent with its ethical legitimacy. For example, one of the major reasons for a new brain-centered definition of death, formulated by the Harvard Committee in 1968 (discussed in Chapter 3), was to facilitate withdrawing LST (Ad hoc Committee 1968). Recognizing that patients diagnosed with irreversible apneic coma are dead would immunize clinicians from charges that they caused the death of these patients by withdrawing treatment. The implication was that if they were not already dead, then stopping treatment would be causing (or seen as causing) death.

The judicial opinion in the Quinlan case (Supreme Court of New Jersey 1976), involving a woman in a permanent vegetative state being maintained in an intensive care unit (ICU), supports this thesis that many doctors were concerned that stopping a respirator could be regarded as causing death: "It seemed to be the consensus not only of the treating physicians but also of the qualified experts who testified in the case, that removal from the respirator would not conform to medical practices, standards and traditions" (56). It would not conform because doing so would arguably be a lethal act causing the patient's death. Indeed, the Court in describing Quinlan's situation observed that "Her life accordingly is sustained by the respirator and tubal feeding, and removal from the respirator *would cause her death* soon, although the time cannot be stated with more precision" (57, italics added). To be sure, the judicial opinion in the Quinlan case is somewhat ambiguous concerning the issue of causing death. On the one hand, in addition to the preceding statement, the Court noted that "[w]e are aware that such termination of treatment would accelerate Karen's death" (73). On the other hand, in the same paragraph of the opinion, it is stated that "[w]e believe that the ensuing death would not be homicide but rather expiration from existing natural causes" (73). This clearly seems inconsistent with the other quotations regarding stopping the ventilator as causing, or accelerating, death. Nevertheless, the Court proceeds to make the important point, which has been neglected in subsequent discussion of end-of-life practices, that "even if it were to be regarded as homicide, it would not be unlawful" (73). Given the finding that the patient had a constitutional "right of privacy" to terminate treatment, the withdrawal of treatment would not "come within the scope of homicide statutes proscribing only the unlawful killing of another" (73).

The court opinion authorized withdrawing the ventilator from Quinlan; however, she remained alive because by the time the opinion was issued her brain injury recovered sufficiently to enable her to breathe spontaneously after being weaned gradually from the ventilator. Because not all patients die after withdrawal of mechanical ventilation does not change the fact that this cessation of treatment does cause death for some patients—that is, for those who are incapable of maintaining adequate respiratory function because of their neurological injury. Additionally, sedation properly administered to relieve suffering following a planned withdrawal of respiratory support further increases the high probability that patients will die as a result. Moreover, withdrawing artificial feeding for patients in a permanent vegetative state, as in the case of Nancy Cruzan, will invariably cause death (if no intervening cause of death occurs).

Although the judicial opinion in Quinlan described withdrawing LST as causing death (though not consistently throughout), by 1997 Justice Rehnquist, writing the majority opinion for the Supreme Court in *Vacco v. Quill* (1997), took the stance that withdrawing LST, in contrast to assisted suicide, does not cause death. He declared that there is a rational distinction between withdrawing LST and assisted suicide: "The distinction comports with fundamental legal principles of causation and intent. First, when a patient refuses life-sustaining treatment, he dies from the underlying fatal disease or pathology; but if a patient ingests lethal medication prescribed by a physician, he is killed by that medication" (425). Perhaps Rehnquist merely meant that as a matter of law withdrawing LST does not count as causing death (i.e., it is not treated as criminal homicide—an issue that we discuss at the end of this chapter); however, the quoted statement more naturally appears to be describing the facts with respect to what causes the patient's death. The stance that withdrawing LST does not cause death became hardened into dogma within medical ethics, and the law, despite being patently contrary to the common-sense conception of causation.

The prevailing view about withdrawing LST has been widely asserted but rarely defended by argument. Therefore, it is worth examining in some detail an argument in its defense by Callahan (1992). "Against common opinion, the argument is sometimes made that there is no moral difference between stopping life-sustaining treatment and more active forms of killing, such as lethal injection. Instead I would contend that the notion that there is no morally significant difference between omission and commission is just wrong" (53). Whether or not there is a morally significant difference between an omission and a commission, each of which is followed by a patient's death, describing stopping LST as an omission is an odd, though not uncommon, characterization. Stopping a ventilator is an active intervention into an ongoing process of sustaining a patient's life by artificial respiration. Turning off the ventilator is no more an omission than is turning off a lamp by pushing a switch.

To be sure, the President's Commission (1983) claimed that there is ambiguity in whether withdrawing mechanical ventilation should be regarded as an act or an omission. "Sometimes deciding whether a particular course involves an act or an omission is less than clear. Stopping a respirator at the request of a competent patient who would have lived with it for a few years but who will die without it in just a few hours is such an ambiguous case. Does the physician omit continuing the treatment or act to disconnect it?" (65–66). We see no such ambiguity. Clearly, the physician first acts to disconnect the respirator. Then it might be said that further respiratory therapy is omitted. But it is the act of turning off the respirator that sets in motion the chain of events leading to the patient's death in a few hours.

Callahan (1992) proceeds to explain why those who view stopping LST as morally equivalent to active euthanasia are wrong: "They are confused, first, when the action of a physician in stopping treatment of a patient with an underlying lethal disease is construed as *causing* death. On the contrary, the physician's omission can only bring about death on the condition that the patient's disease will kill him in the absence of treatment. . . But it confuses reality and moral judgment to see an omitted action as having the same causal status as one that directly kills. A lethal injection will kill both a healthy person and a sick person. Turn off the machine on me, a healthy person, and nothing will happen. It will only, in contrast, bring the life of a sick person to an end because of an underlying fatal disease" (53).

Callahan errs here by failing to recognize the distinction, central to the common-sense conception of causation, between what is identified as the cause of an event and associated conditions necessary for the cause to produce its effect. The underlying lethal disease or injury (e.g., the spinal cord injury and resulting quadriplegia of the patient considered above) is no different, in principle, from underlying necessary conditions that are present in all cases of causation. Turning off the ignition of a car causes it to stop running and pushing a light switch causes the lamp to go out. In both of these cases there are underlying conditions that are necessary for the cause to produce its effect: the ignition must be wired to the engine and the switch must be wired to the lamp, just as the ventilator switch is wired to the ventilator. Likewise, turning the ignition key will start the car only if the battery is working.

Consider the following case. A careless hiker throws a lit cigarette into the woods, causing a forest fire. The act wouldn't have caused the fire if the woods were wet, rather than extremely dry; nor would the fire have spread widely if the wind wasn't blowing. But neither of these underlying conditions negates the common-sense judgment that throwing the lit cigarette into the woods caused the forest fire. We don't say that the dry conditions or the wind caused the forest fire. The patient's underlying medical condition is (to some extent) analogous to these underlying conditions necessary for the fire to start and spread. We also distinguish between causes and conditions in common medical situations. Influenza will make a healthy young person sick for a relatively short period of time, after which health is restored. A frail elderly person, however, may die from influenza. What leaves the former intact causes death to the latter, just as turning off a ventilator connected to a healthy person in Callahan's example has no impact on this person's ability to breathe, but turning it off for a ventilator-dependent quadriplegic, contra Callahan, causes death. The fact that turning off the ventilator results in death only for patients with an underlying medical condition that makes them incapable of breathing spontaneously is fully consistent with the fact that the withdrawal of treatment causes death.

There is, however, an element of disanalogy between the case of withdrawing LST and the forest fire case. The dry woods and the wind do not have the power by themselves to cause a fire. The patient's disease does have the power to cause death *if* unchecked by LST. It doesn't follow that the disease by itself is the cause of the patient's death; for if the LST had not been withdrawn, the patient would have continued to live. Stopping the ventilator sets in motion the causal process that leads to the ventilator-dependent patient's death at the time when it occurred.

Causation and Common Sense

In characterizing withdrawing LST, we have been appealing to a common-sense conception of causation. It may be objected, however, that we have failed to recognize that people commonly make causal judgments regarding human action within a normative context in which "cause" is used to assign moral responsibility. The empirical literature on the way that people determine causation demonstrates that these judgments are often affected by moral considerations relating to responsibility, blame, intention, and motivations. For example, if a bad outcome was intended by an agent, or the agent's behavior was connected to a morally objectionable motivation, people are more likely to judge that the agent caused the outcome than if it was unintended or connected to a good motivation (Alicke 1992; Lagnado and Channon 2008). Consider again Brock's thought experiment designed to rebut the conventional wisdom about causing death in medicine, which we deployed above. The "enemy" who turns off the ventilator thereby kills the patient, whereas the doctor who orders the ventilator to be stopped in response to the patient's or surrogate's refusal of treatment allegedly merely allows the patient to die. Brock argued that if the former causes death, then so must the latter, because it is the very same act in both cases. Nevertheless, based on the empirical literature on causation, we can anticipate that if people were asked to judge on a scale of 1 to 10 the extent to which the agent caused the patient's death in these two cases, they would report much higher scores in the enemy scenario than in the doctor scenario. Indeed, people might generally endorse the prevailing view in medical ethics that in withdrawing LST, when justified, clinicians are not causing death.

How, then, can we be correct in arguing that on a common-sense view of causation the prevailing view is false? Common sense does not necessarily coincide with what most people would judge. Furthermore, we are adopting a "critical common-sense" perspective, aimed at deploying the conception of causation operative in ordinary life but free of biases that may interfere with causal judgments. Because we can, and often do, distinguish between causation of an outcome and moral responsibility and/or blame for causing the outcome, there exist grounds for judging that causal judgments can be biased by moral considerations, even when these biases are widespread. An "ideal observer" impartially examining a scenario of human action in light of our common-sense conception of causation would make causal judgments independent of moral considerations. This is the bias-free standard to which we appeal.

Clearly, in many scientific disciplines causal judgments regarding human action are made without any reference to moral considerations. Medicine is centrally concerned with causal judgments about the outcomes of treatment interventions, which involve clinicians prescribing or administering treatments and making inferences about the contribution of these treatments to either beneficial outcomes or adverse events. Moral considerations are irrelevant to the causal judgments. It is worth noting, however, that these causal judgments are highly liable to bias, as doctors and their patients naturally are disposed to judge that when patients get better after taking a treatment, the treatment was the cause of the improvement. To overcome the fallacy of *post hoc ergo propter hoc*, randomized controlled trials are employed to detect causation. We argue below that ordinary judgments of causation are liable to a different sort of bias derived from moral considerations.

Despite the tendency of people to conflate moral responsibility and causation in actual judgments, it is clear that these concepts are logically distinct. We often are able to make causal judgments regarding bad outcomes, even in emotionally charged situations, that are independent of moral considerations. Consider the following cases. First, a young man suffering from schizophrenia stabs his mother under the influence of a command hallucination and delusionary beliefs. We don't hold him legally or morally responsible for his mother's death, because of his insanity, but we still say that he killed his mother. Second, an automobile driver going at the speed limit runs over a child who has bolted into the street. There was no way that the driver could avoid hitting the child, who dies as the result of the accident. Although we don't hold the driver responsible for wrongdoing, we say that the child was killed by the motor vehicle—i.e., the driver caused the death of the child. In both these cases we attribute the act that caused death to the agent, even though we don't hold the agent morally responsible for causing the death. In the medical context, everyone agrees that giving a patient a lethal injection causes the patient's death, including those who support the ethics of active euthanasia. Hence the causal judgment is independent of ascribing moral responsibility for an alleged wrongful act, for active euthanasia is not necessarily wrong. In all these cases of human action, there is a morally independent fact of the matter of whether an active intervention causes a given outcome.

It seems all the more clear, when moral considerations are set aside, that withdrawing LST causes death. The clinician who turns off the ventilator (or orders that it be turned off) knows what he or she is doing and knows the probable consequences of the act. No physical or mental compulsion forces the clinician's hand. Absent commitment to the norm that clinicians must not (intentionally) cause the death of their patients, it seems undeniable that withdrawing LST contributes causally to patients' deaths.

Omissions

We argued above that it is a mistake to view withdrawing LST as an omission. This mistake, however, is central to understanding the prevailing view that withdrawing LST does not cause death. Accordingly, it is important to examine the common-sense thinking regarding the causal role of omissions. It has generally been thought in the philosophical literature that causation involves a relationship between events. How can an omission—the absence of something—which is certainly not an event, count as a cause? Although this may be a puzzle from a metaphysical perspective, causal explanation by reference to omission or absence is commonplace not only in ordinary life but in medical science. What caused the plants to wither and die during a drought? The absence of rain or the lack of human watering provides a sufficient explanation. This is not just a matter of folk psychology. Scientific explanation of many diseases is traced to the absence of biologically needed chemicals, vitamins, proteins, etc. Scurvy, for example, is caused by the absence of vitamin C.

In the case of human action, omissions often are properly judged to be causal when an agent has a duty or responsibility to do the omitted act, and not otherwise. This creates a curious asymmetry with causal judgments that apply to active interventions, in which causation is, or should be, understood as distinct from moral responsibility. Thus, parents who fail to feed their infant children are judged to have caused their children's death. A neighbor who is aware that the children are seriously malnourished may be held responsible for not reporting this to established authorities but wouldn't be considered to have caused the children's death by virtue of omitting to feed them. In accordance with this logic of omissions, in the medical context, omissions to provide treatment are generally judged to cause a patient's death only when there is a duty to treat. For example, not intubating a patient does not cause the patient to die from respiratory failure if there is no duty to treat (because, say, the patient refused it in an advance directive, it would be futile, more burdensome than beneficial, or only prolong the process of dying). But if a doctor fails to provide LST for a patient in need of care who has not refused treatment, because the doctor wants the patient to die (for some illicit reason) or because of negligence, then the omission causes (or contributes to causing) the patient's death.

Omissions of human action may be causal, however, when there is no duty to do what is omitted. Some terminally or incurably ill patients decide to hasten death by refusing to eat and drink. This is morally justifiable when based on self-determination and a reasonable judgment of personal well-being (in contrast, for example, to a refusal to eat by a young person suffering from anorexia). In these circumstances the patient has no duty to eat or drink, yet it makes sense to describe the cause of death as dehydration and/or starvation owing to the refusal to eat and drink. What makes the omission causal is deviation from what is normal and therefore expected.

The error in judging that withdrawing LST does not cause death might be diagnosed, in part, as mistakenly treating the active intervention of stopping LST as if it were an omission of treatment. If it were an omission, and assuming no duty to treat, then stopping LST would not cause death. Because, however, withdrawing LST is something that clinicians do—an active intervention, not an omission—the fact that a doctor has a duty to comply with a patient's refusal of treatment has no logical bearing on the correct causal attribution for the outcome. There is a sense in which the doctor has no choice, from a moral perspective, but to stop LST when a competent patient has refused treatment. But this doesn't change the fact that turning off the ventilator is a voluntary act that causes death; it makes the difference between the patient's continued living and the occurrence of death at the time it occurs.

More broadly, the error in the prevailing view derives from *moral bias*, which we discuss in some detail below. Causation and culpability for harm or wrongdoing are logically distinct concepts, at least with respect to active human interventions. Setting aside the traditional norm that doctors must not kill, withdrawing LST would be discerned clearly as causing death in many instances. However, commitment to this established norm drives the false judgment that clinicians are not causing death when they routinely and appropriately withdraw LST. This normative commitment operates as a moral bias—a motivated deviation from the truth—that turns withdrawing LST into an omission that merely allows the patient to die a natural death, despite the fact that the withdrawal of treatment is an active intervention that hastens the occurrence of death, in some cases making it occur much sooner than it otherwise would absent the withdrawal. This moral bias obscures the fact that causing death is a routine feature of contemporary medicine. Moreover, causing death by means of withdrawing LST is an ethically legitimate practice, grounded in the values of patient self-determination and well-being. It follows that the traditional norm that doctors must not kill needs to be modified.

INTENTION AND DOUBLE EFFECT

Some commentators will no doubt respond that we are much too hasty in claiming that this traditional norm should be modified. They will concede that withdrawing LST causes death. However, the traditional norm should be understood as prohibiting clinicians from *intentionally* causing the death of patients. Causing death may be legitimate in a range of circumstances in which it is merely foreseen as likely to occur by medical intervention or by the active termination of ongoing treatment but is not intended. In this regard, practitioners and ethicists appeal to the doctrine of *double effect* to justify withdrawing LST.

Appeal to the double effect in this context has a long-standing pedigree, going back over 50 years, to the early stage of facing the ethical issues posed by life-sustaining medical technology. In 1957, an anesthesiologist asked Pope Pius XII for guidance with respect to the ethics of withdrawing mechanical ventilation in the case of hopelessly ill patients. According to the Pope, "[e]ven when it causes the arrest of circulation, the interruption of attempts at resuscitation is never more than an indirect cause of the cessation of life, and one must apply in this case the principle of double effect" (Pope Pius XII 1957a). It is clear from the context of the Pope's statement that by "interruption of attempts at resuscitation" he meant stopping the ventilator. Whatever might have been meant by "indirect cause," the role of withdrawing LST in causing death is definitely affirmed. Indeed, it must be affirmed for the doctrine of double effect to operate.

The doctrine of double effect is a traditional stance in Catholic moral theology, which has also assumed a prominent role in secular medical ethics, most frequently in justifying high doses of pain-relieving medication that risk hastening the death of a terminally ill patient. (We discuss this latter context in Chapter 2.) In general, the doctrine is invoked to justify acts that have both a good and a bad or harmful effect. Beauchamp and Childress (2009, 162–163) summarize the four key conditions for the double effect as follows:

1. *The nature of the act.* The act must be good, or at least morally neutral, independent of its consequences.
2. *The agent's intention.* The agent intends only the good effect, not the bad effect. The bad effect can be foreseen, tolerated, and permitted, but it must not be intended.
3. *The distinction between means and effects.* The bad effect must not be a means to the good effect. If the good effect were the causal result of the bad effect, the agent would intend the bad effect in pursuit of the good effect.
4. *Proportionality between the good effect and the bad effect.* The good effect must outweigh the bad effect. That is, the bad effect is permissible only if a proportionate reason compensates for permitting the foreseen bad effect.

Applied to withdrawing LST, the good effect can be variously understood as respecting patient self-determination and/or promoting well-being by removing a burdensome treatment. The bad effect is death caused by withdrawing treatment. The intent of the clinician must be to produce the good effect, not to cause death. In the case of active euthanasia by lethal injection, which also may be undertaken to respect self-determination and to promote patient well-being by putting an end to intolerable suffering, the good effect, assuming that there is a good effect, is produced by means of the bad effect of death caused by the lethal injection. In contrast, in withdrawing LST the bad effect of death is alleged not to be the means of producing the good effects of respecting self-determination and removing burdensome and unwanted treatment, which are produced by stopping the treatment. Finally, in view of the situation of the patient, there is a proportionate reason for producing the foreseen but not intended effect of death.

A vast interpretive and critical literature has developed regarding the ethical significance of the double effect doctrine (McIntyre 2009). We will confine our attention here to a few key points pertinent to withdrawing LST. First, it begs the question of characterizing death as a bad or harmful effect in this context. When death puts an end to the suffering and burdens of a mode of existence sustained by medical technology, it may be seen by the patient as a (relatively) good outcome. The phrase "a fate worse than death," and describing pneumonia traditionally as "the old man's friend," suggest tragic or intolerable states of human existence for which death offers relief and release. As Beauchamp and Childress (2009) observe, "[o]ften in dispute is whether death is good or bad for a particular person, and nothing in the RDE [rule of double effect] settles this dispute" (165). When death is perceived as better than continued living in the unfortunate circumstances faced by the hopelessly ill patient tethered to medical technology, then the double effect doctrine has no purchase, unless death is viewed (unreasonably) as an objective harm under all circumstances. Whereas death typically is the greatest harm that can befall human beings, this is not universally the case. A default judgment about the harm or badness of death will often not hold up in the context of end-of-life decisions. Accordingly, in many cases when withdrawing LST is ethically legitimate, the doctrine of double effect lacks traction from the outset.

Second, the claim that the agent responsible for withdrawing LST does not intend to cause death is empirically suspect in many cases. Moreover, it is ethically dubious that clinicians should never intend to cause death when it is legitimate to withdraw LST. These points are important irrespective of commitment to the double effect, as many consider it always wrong to intend to cause the death of an innocent person. Consider the case of John, a motorcycle enthusiast. At age 50 he experienced a serious accident that left him quadriplegic and dependent on a ventilator to breathe. After rehabilitative treatment, John returns home and lives for 3 years with the help of family and employed caretakers.

Over time he finds his situation intolerable. John decides that he no longer wants to continue living owing to complete dependence on others for activities of daily living and the associated absence of privacy. He asks to be admitted to the hospital where he was treated after the accident in order to have his home ventilator withdrawn and receive palliative care needed to die peacefully. A clinician who views John's plan as reasonable given his circumstances, values, and preferences, and is prepared to help by withdrawing his ventilator, may actually and legitimately intend not only to respect John's autonomous choice but to cause death in order to realize his plan.

Brody (1996) notes that the claim that clinicians do not intend death in cases of withdrawing LST is inconsistent with his experience as an ethics consultant in the clinical setting. "In many cases of withholding or withdrawing therapy, it is the continued existence of the patient in the condition in which they are in which is found burdensome, not the treatment itself. 'Mama wouldn't have wanted to live this way' is the common refrain, and withholdings or withdrawings of therapy are undertaken in response to that refrain. The death may be the intended end for which the decision is made, or, more plausibly, the intended means to avoid the continued suffering and indignity of living that way. It is certainly not a mere foreseen side effect" (99). This point tells against both the second and third condition of the doctrine of double effect. Not only is the patient's death often intended in legitimate withdrawing of LST, death may be the means to avoid an intolerable continued existence.

Recent empirical evidence indicates that many physicians, at least in Europe, acknowledge an intention to cause death when withdrawing life support. A large-scale survey of end-of-life decisions in six European countries (Belgium, Denmark, Italy, the Netherlands, Sweden, and Switzerland) demonstrated that a majority of physicians reported an explicit intention to hasten death when mechanical respiration (66%) and dialysis (69%) were withdrawn (Bosshard et al. 2006). (Intending to hasten death is the same as intending to cause death, as hastening death causes death to occur earlier than it otherwise would.) Discussing their findings, the authors state that "[t]he data presented in this paper clearly show that the view that withholding or withdrawing treatment means allowing patients to die, even though not intending them to do so, is untenable from an empirical point of view." Additionally, they observe that "in the context of withholding and withdrawing treatment there is a great divergence between the traditional moral rule and today's medical practice."

We do not claim, however, that whenever life-sustaining treatment is withdrawn clinicians necessarily intend to cause death. Certainly, if the intention is to determine whether the patient can be weaned from a ventilator, as in the Quinlan case following the court decision, there is no such intent. Additionally, in the case of terminally ill patients who are likely to die in a short period of time regardless of continued life-sustaining treatment, the primary intention of clinicians often may be to remove a burdensome and unwanted impediment to a peaceful death, foreseeing that doing so is likely to hasten death. In some cases, clinicians may personally disapprove of the patient's decision to stop LST but comply in view of the patient's right to refuse treatment. In these cases the clinicians would not be intending to cause death, though the LST would be stopped intentionally in response to a patient's refusal. Nevertheless, it is important to recognize that in practice it is often not easy to distinguish between what is intended and what is foreseen but not intended. Moreover, as Quill (1993) has argued, clinical intentions relating to end-of-life decisions are often multiple and ambiguous—a fact that is obscured by the strictures of the double effect doctrine.

Like the view that withdrawing LST does not cause death, the doctrine of double effect as applied to this domain introduces or reinforces moral biases that skew accurate characterization of routine medical practice. Both perspectives bias the description of medical practice at the end of life, leading to mistaken accounts of causation and intention. In both perspectives the moral bias is driven by commitment to the questionable (absolute) norm that clinicians must not kill.

RESPONSIBILITY FOR CAUSING DEATH

According to the prevailing perspective in medical ethics, clinicians are not morally responsible for causing the death of patients in withdrawing LST precisely because they do not cause death by means of this practice. When this perspective on causation is seen to be erroneous and a product of moral bias, then so is the prevailing understanding of moral responsibility. It is important to understand what is meant by "moral responsibility." We are morally responsible for voluntary acts that can be attributed to us, whether right or wrong. Specifically, a clinician is morally responsible for causing a patient's death by withdrawing a ventilator when this life-terminating act can be attributed from a moral perspective to the clinician. Is causing the death something that the physician did voluntarily and knowingly, such that it can be attributed to him? We are morally responsible for what we intend to do, or do knowingly, or do negligently. It follows that clinicians are responsible for causing the death of patients by withdrawing life support, regardless of whether we agree with the claim that death is intended in many, but not necessarily all, of these cases. Moral responsibility for causing death does not equate to culpability for wrong doing, unless it is presumed that it is always wrong to do so. Death-causing treatment withdrawals can be right or wrong acts depending on the circumstances, including critically the informed consent (or refusal) of competent patients or legally authorized surrogate decision makers.

In withdrawing life-sustaining treatment, responsibility for causing death is shared by patients or surrogates and clinicians. Indeed, the primary responsibility rests with the patient, or surrogate deciding on behalf of the patient. This prior authorization for treatment withdrawal is a morally necessary condition for clinicians (justifiably) taking responsibility for withdrawing life support and thus for causing the death that ensues (Miller et al. 2010).

MORAL BIAS

We have described our claim that the prevailing view in medical ethics of withdrawing LST involves a series of moral biases relating to causation, intention, and responsibility, which are driven by commitment to the traditional norm that doctors must not kill their patients. In this section, we offer a more general account of moral bias to further explain our diagnosis of the prevailing views in medical ethics about the withdrawal of LST. To have a bias is to make judgments that deviate form the truth based on a psychological motive or reason. The bias is motivated. A psychological disposition interferes with perceiving the truth. A moral bias is a *motivated* false belief about human conduct that serves a *legitimating* function.

Some generic features of situations faced by health professionals and investigators give rise to moral bias. Professional practices regarded as legitimate sometimes conflict, or are in tension, with established professional, ethical, or legal norms. Professionals faced with these conflicts find themselves in a state of "cognitive dissonance" (Tavris and Aronson 2007). They want to continue performing the practices in question, but they also want to uphold these conflicting norms. How can this be done without patent inconsistency or incoherence? Moral biases conveniently eliminate or ease the tension. We have characterized the prevailing view that withdrawing life-sustaining treatment merely allows the patient to die but does not cause death as a moral bias. This moral bias brings established medical practices at the end of life in line with the established norm that doctors must not kill. Absent this moral bias, commitment to the established norm would make withdrawing life-sustaining treatment, understood as a death-causing act, unethical. This psychological dynamic, which produces a morally biased account of a practice, may operate not only for practitioners but also for ethicists who are appraising the practice.

The moral biases relating to end-of-life practices are complex and deep in a number of respects. First, they are deeply entrenched in the attitudes of practitioners and in medical ethics. Second, they involve the intersection between factual beliefs, interpretation and application of basic concepts (causation, intention, and death), and established moral norms. Third, they are deep psychologically. Traditionally the healing role has been understood as incompatible ethically with causing death deliberately or knowingly: hence, the norm that doctors must not kill. In fact, the power of medicine to sustain life by means of technological interventions, when these interventions are not able to cure the underlying life-threatening conditions, goes hand in hand with the power to cause death when these treatments are withdrawn. The positive side is affirmed, though not without disquiet about sustaining life when it may be more burdensome than beneficial to the patient. The negative, flip side that withdrawing LST causes death is denied. For if it were affirmed, clinicians and ethicists would have to face the power of contemporary medicine to cause death legitimately, indicating the need to modify the traditional normative commitment that prohibits causing death. Even when withdrawing LST is recognized as causing death, the conflict with the traditional norm that doctors must not kill has been masked by claiming that death is merely foreseen but not intended. In both cases, moral biases distort an accurate accounting of the facts relating to contemporary medical practice.

Moral biases within biomedicine are by no means limited to end-of-life practices. The ethics of clinical research also reflects moral biases. It has been argued that clinical trials are characterized by a "therapeutic orientation," which treats them as essentially a form of medical care governed by the ethics of the fiduciary doctor–patient relationship (Miller and Brody 2003; Miller and Rosenstein 2003). This obscures the way in which clinical trials differ in ethically significant ways from personalized medical care—specifically with respect to their purpose, characteristic methods, and way in which risks to patient-subjects are justified. Commitment to the ethics of the doctor–patient relationship creates a morally biased account of the design and conduct of clinical trials. This is reflected in the ethically dubious norm of clinical equipoise, which is intended to make clinical trials consistent with the traditional ethics of medical care.

Moral biases operate in accordance with an underlying "logic": This is how things are so that they can be as they ought to be. Allegiance to a general norm or a particular judgment about what ought to be done dictates the (erroneous) description of facts so that they are consistent with the general norm or particular moral judgment. The "logic" of moral bias may be seen, in effect, as a reversal of the so-called "naturalistic fallacy." Ethical reasoning often moves from factual premises to normative conclusions; and this is held by some, but certainly not all, moral philosophers to be an illicit inference. With respect to moral bias, views about the way things ought (or ought not) to be dictate judgments about how they in fact are, so as to achieve coherence between conduct and established norms. To be sure, clinicians and ethicists do not derive the claim that the routine practice of withdrawing life-sustaining practice merely allows patients to die as a logical inference from the norm that doctors must not kill their patients. Rather, they believe (or at least espouse the belief) that, as a matter of fact, turning off a ventilator does not cause the death of patients who are unable to sustain adequate spontaneous respiratory function. We suggest that they hold this false belief because of their commitment to the established norm. Although in some cases moral biases may involve logical fallacies, the diagnosis of moral biases that we are suggesting is essentially psychological. Commitment to established norms and to practices that in fact conflict with them creates "cognitive dissonance," which is resolved by means of invoking morally biased beliefs about the practices in question.

Moral biases not only are invoked to legitimate practices by means of false beliefs; as suggested above, they also serve to hide, or divert attention from, the truth about these practices, which might call their legitimacy into question. Describing withdrawing life-sustaining treatment as merely allowing patients to die a natural death from the underlying medical condition that is being treated by medical technology hides the fact that stopping these treatments causes the patient's death and thus conflicts with conventional medical ethics. In describing moral biases as hiding the truth, we do not imply any overt intention to do so, although this may be operative in some circumstances. Moral biases hide the truth about underlying incoherence between practices and norms, not only for those who engage in the practices in questions; they also hide the truth from patients, ethicists, and the public.

Moral bias is a natural psychological tendency to which all of us are liable. In truth, the way the world works often doesn't conform to the way we think it should; accordingly, when this lack of congruity matters to us, we are often motivated to adopt false beliefs so that the conflict between "fact" and value is made to disappear. In other words, people are often motivated to endorse false beliefs so that they can view themselves and their conduct as appropriate in light of established norms. In view of the psychological function of moral biases, especially when deeply rooted, there may be considerable resistance to acknowledging their existence.

Our appeal to moral bias faces a theoretical objection. We have claimed that it is a matter of *fact* that withdrawing LST causes death. How can we be confident that this is a fact, especially in view of the prevailing perspective that denies it? Facts are not independent of interpretative theories, which may be contested (Tauber 2009). It may be further objected that our account of causation free of "moral bias" relies on an uncritical distinction between fact and value, casting in doubt whether we can meaningfully tease apart the facts about human causation from value judgments relating to the "facts." Moreover, we have conceded that in the case of omissions, people normally and properly assign causation in light of agents' duties and responsibilities. If we are deploying moral values in assigning causation with respect to omissions, then why not with respect to human acts, especially those sort of acts, such as withdrawing LST, that involve stopping an intervention and omitting to restart it?

This is not the place for a philosophical account of facts and the relationship between facts and values. And in any case, any account of these disputed philosophical issues that we might propose would be less likely to secure conviction than our argument that withdrawing LST causes death. We describe the fact that withdrawing LST causes death not as some brute or naked fact about the way the world works but as a reasonable inference from the implicit theory of causation embedded in common sense. Our view thus stands or falls on the validity of our application of the common-sense conception of causation—an admittedly complex but familiar conception—to the practice of withdrawing LST. As noted above, our understanding of causation is a critical or purified version of common sense, which explains human actions independent of the normative assessment of those actions. We ask the reader to examine and reflect on withdrawing LST, bearing in mind the distinction between causation and culpability. Although we advance various arguments supporting our position, ultimately there is no proof other than appealing to an unbiased judgment that an ideal observer would make.

We submit, furthermore, that despite the conventional view that withdrawing LST merely allows patients to die, it often *feels* like active causation to clinicians and observers—an act that sets in motion a causal process leading to death. And we propose a diagnostic hypothesis to explain the denial of the fact that this feeling reflects. Commitment to the norm that doctors must not kill turns the act of causing death by means of withdrawing LST into an omission of treatment that merely allows the patient to die. This stance constitutes what we call moral bias. It is a moral bias not in the sense that it leads to an incorrect moral evaluation of withdrawing LST. Rather, it distorts and hides the facts about the causal connection between treatment withdrawal and death. It does this in service of immunizing clinicians from the force of the established norm that prohibits them from killing (causing death of) their patients. This moral bias also gives comfort to family members who must make decisions about withdrawing treatment for incompetent patients and who do not want to see themselves as responsible for causing the death of their loved ones.

Should we purge medical ethics of moral biases surrounding end-of-life decisions? Because these moral biases serve psychological and social functions, should they be exposed and should efforts be made to eliminate them? These are basic questions for the inquiry we are pursuing here. The moral biases infecting the prevailing perspective in medical ethics on withdrawing LST may be seen as having promoted moral progress by making clinicians, ethicists, patients, family members, and society comfortable with morally challenging and emotionally troubling end-of-life practices. As mentioned above, expert testimony provided in the 1976 Quinlan case indicated that withdrawing LST such as a respirator was considered contrary to the practices, standards, and traditions of the medical profession. Stevens, in her revisionary history of bioethics in America, has disputed this, claiming that doctors commonly turned off respirators for hopelessly ill patients but were reluctant to state this publicly in a court of law, owing to concerns about potential legal liability (Stevens 2000, 113). In any case, regardless of when withdrawing LST became routine practice, it came out of the closet as the result of the Quinlan case. Over the next decade or so, it had become publicly, and almost universally, regarded as ethically legitimate; subsequently, it was recognized by the U.S. Supreme Court as grounded in a fundamental constitutional right.

From a historical perspective, it is difficult to see how this moral progress could have been achieved without the prevailing views relating to causation, intention, and responsibility that, according to our analysis, reflect moral biases. The President's Commission's report, *Deciding to Forego Life-Sustaining Treatment*, includes a remarkable paragraph in support of this diagnosis (without any appeal to the concept of moral bias), which we quote in full.

"Yet in health care, and especially with critically or terminally ill patients, it is common to make decisions that one knows risk shortening patient's lives and that sometimes turn out to do so. As a result, there is a strong motivation to interpret the actions decided upon and carried out, especially if by people other than the patient, as something other than acts of killing. Thus, the concerned parties very much want these to be regarded as cases of "allowing to die" (rather than "killing"), of "not prolonging the dying process" (instead of "hastening death"), or of "failing to stop a disease from causing death" (rather than "someone's action was the cause of death"). Consequently, these distinctions, while often conceptually unclear and of dubious moral importance in themselves, are useful in facilitating acceptance of sound decisions that would otherwise meet unwarranted resistance. They help people involved to understand, in ways acceptable to them, their proper role in implementing decisions to forego life-sustaining treatment" (President's Commission 1983:71).

According to our analysis, all of the preferred descriptions of end-of-life practices in the preceding paragraph reflect false or skewed descriptions reflecting moral bias, driven by commitment to an unwarranted absolute norm that clinicians must not (intentionally) cause the death of their patients. Nevertheless, shouldn't these moral biases be preserved in view of the professional and social functions that they serve, eloquently described by the President's Commission? The very same question will arise in light of our critical analysis in subsequent chapters of prevailing views relating to organ donation and the determination of death.

It is premature to attempt a comprehensive answer. At this stage we simply suggest a few reasons for challenging the various moral biases associated with the prevailing perspective relating to withdrawing LST. Because they reflect false factual judgments and erroneous use of basic concepts such as causation and intention, both honesty and commitment to rational coherence in the development of medical ethics argue in favor of eliminating these moral biases. In the realm of truth-seeking scholarship, they can play no legitimate role. Moreover, as we shall argue in the next chapter, these particular moral biases skew the ethical appraisal of active euthanasia by supporting a misguided ethical bright line between forgoing LST and active intervention to cause death by means of lethal injection. As such, they have important practical implications, insofar as maintaining the prohibition of active euthanasia deprives suffering patients of a potentially legitimate means of a humane and dignified death. In the next chapter we take up the questions of how active euthanasia relates to withdrawing LST, whether it can be ethically justified, and whether it is desirable as a matter of policy to legalize a practice of lethal injection by physicians under specified ethical and regulatory constraints.

This objection might be pressed further. Granted that moral progress in withdrawing LST depended on seeing this as merely allowing patients to die and not as causing death, isn't this moral progress at risk of being turned back if it became widely believed or publicly acknowledged that withdrawing treatment causes death? We view it as highly unlikely that patients, family members, and clinicians would refuse to stop life support. Basic to medical ethics is the goal of relieving suffering and refraining from administering treatments for which the burdens or harms are disproportionate to the benefits. Moreover, the right to refuse medical treatment has strong support in the law—a right that is not logically grounded on any view of causation or intention on the part of clinicians. Although facing the facts about causation and intention might create moral discomfort for clinicians, in view of the conflict between these facts and traditional medical ethics, clinicians would remain obliged to respect the rights of patients to refuse LST.

Setting aside the issues of preserving moral progress and promoting moral comfort, the implications of endorsing moral biases should be faced. Think of how medical ethics is being construed if it needs to rely on falsehood to guide medical practice. Can ethics as a reflective and rational discipline be grounded in a denial of reality? How can it command respect if it flies in the face of the facts? Perhaps there are truths that are too hard to bear. Perhaps medical ethics, especially in its practical deployment, must be based on false beliefs about medical practice. But if so, the burden of proof is on our critics to demonstrate that this is so.

WITHDRAWING TREATMENT AND HOMICIDE

A final practical objection to our position that withdrawing LST causes death deserves attention. Doesn't our position imply that withdrawing LST would fall under the jurisdiction of the criminal law? Consent to be killed is not recognized as a defense to homicide. We suggest two responses to this objection. First, as stated by the court in *Quinlan*, the criminal law prohibits unlawful (or wrongful) homicide. Patients have a legal right to refuse treatment, grounded in a constitutional liberty right and the common law right of bodily integrity, which makes treatment without consent a form of battery. Therefore, homicide statutes have no application to cases of withdrawing LST that come within the scope of the patient's right to refuse treatment. Second, what counts as causation in the law is not the same as causation in fact. Thus, the law need not treat withdrawing LST as causing death. This response essentially amounts to adopting a transparent legal fiction, which may be justified by the social purpose of exempting clinicians from legal liability when they are practicing medicine competently with respect to withdrawing LST and are respecting patients' rights. We will address the issue of criminal liability in more detail in Chapter 7 in the context of discussing a legal fictions approach to vital organ donation.

2

Active Euthanasia

In contemporary medicine, patients frequently die following a decision, either to withhold or to withdraw treatment. Physician-assisted suicide (PAS) by prescribing lethal medication is legal in Switzerland and in the United States in Oregon and Washington. In the Netherlands and Belgium, the law permits voluntary active euthanasia by a physician's lethal injection. These different ways to die by decision fall along a spectrum of causal involvement of clinicians in the patient's death. If there is no duty to treat, withholding life-sustaining medical treatment (LST) does not cause a patient's death; the attending clinicians stand by and the patient is allowed to die from the progression of a terminal condition. As we argued in the preceding chapter, withdrawing LST causes death, typically in conjunction with the underlying medical condition. In the case of assisted suicide, the clinician provides the patient with the means to cause death, with the decision whether to activate that means left up to the patient. Finally, in active euthanasia the clinician induces death by injecting lethal medication. Are there any ethically significant differences between these ways of causing a patient's death? In this chapter we will focus predominantly on active euthanasia rather than assisted suicide; essentially the same ethical considerations apply to both practices but are brought into bolder relief with reference to the former.

BRIGHT LINES

In 1988, *The Journal of the American Medical Association* (JAMA) published an article by four distinguished physician-ethicists with the title, "Doctors Must Not Kill" (Gaylin et al. 1988). It was written in response to the publication in JAMA of an anonymous report allegedly by a gynecological resident who gave his hospitalized patient dying of cancer a lethal injection of morphine in response to her request, "Let's get this over with." By anyone's standards, the ethics of active euthanasia in this particular case was dubious at best, yet the authors of the critical commentary took advantage of the occasion to issue a general statement about active euthanasia. "[T]he resident violated one of the first and most hallowed canons of medical ethics: doctors must not kill. Generations of physicians and commentators on medical ethics have understood and held fast to the distinction between ceasing useless treatment (or allowing to die) and active, willful taking of life; at least since the Oath of Hippocrates, Western medicine has regarded the killing of patients, even on request, as a profound violation of the deepest meaning of the medical vocation" (2139).

As this statement indicates, the issue of active euthanasia is ancient. The Hippocratic Oath declares, "I will neither give a deadly drug to anybody if asked for it, nor will I make a suggestion to this effect" (Kass 1985, 229). However, the advent of life-sustaining technology has transformed the debate over this issue, raising the question of how active euthanasia compares from a moral perspective with withdrawing LST. Medical ethics has traditionally drawn a bright line between withholding and withdrawing treatment, on the one hand, and both assisted suicide and active euthanasia, on the other. The former is permitted; the latter is prohibited. According to the prevailing view, discussed in Chapter 1, physicians merely allow the patient to die when withholding or withdrawing treatment. If there is no duty to treat, physicians are not regarded as causing death and/or death is not intended. In the case of active euthanasia, by contrast, all agree that the clinician causes and intends to cause the patient's death. With respect to causation and intention, it is less clear why assisted suicide falls on the "bad side" of the bright line. For the physician does not cause the patient's death. Nor is it clear that the physician intends the patient's death. The intent, rather, is to supply the patient with the means of causing his or her own death.

Causation and intention have been regarded as key factors supporting the bright line between withdrawing LST and active euthanasia. In Chapter 1 we argued that clinicians cause death in withdrawing LST and frequently intend to cause death. When moral biases are stripped away from the practice of withdrawing LST, the bright line appears to dim, if not become extinguished entirely. If clinicians do not merely allow patients to die but cause death in withdrawing LST and often intend to do so, what defines the bright line? On what basis is withdrawing LST justified but active euthanasia (always) unethical? Moreover, the ethical considerations that support withdrawing LST—respecting patient self-determination and promoting personal well-being by relieving suffering— also support active euthanasia, especially in response to the request of a competent patient (Brock 1992). The bright line appears to be nothing more than an illusion produced by moral bias, driven by commitment to the established norm that doctors must not kill.

Another ethical bright line is drawn between palliative care that relieves pain and discomfort, on the one hand, and lethal treatment aimed at ending the patient's life, on the other. According to conventional medical ethics, it is ethical to risk hastening death by administering pain-relieving medications, provided that the clinician's plan is to relieve pain and suffering, not to cause death. Indeed, as a last resort, sedation to unconsciousness pending death, including withholding nutrition and hydration, is considered medically and ethically appropriate (Quill et al. 2009). Practitioners and ethicists appeal to the doctrine of double effect to define the bright line between legitimate palliative care and illegitimate active euthanasia. Relieving suffering is the good effect, and causing death is the bad effect. As long as the clinician intends the former but not the latter, it is appropriate to risk hastening death by administering medication. A known lethal regimen or overdose of medication must not be the means to relieve suffering. However, relief of suffering is ethically imperative, making it a proportional rationale for risking hastening death.

This bright line is also highly dubious both empirically and ethically. Clinical intentions are apt to be ambiguous in end-of-life care, making it often difficult, if not impossible, to discern whether a terminally ill patient's treatment falls on the "right" side of the bright line. To be sure, some drug regimens are inherently lethal, such as potassium chloride or the combination of neuromuscular relaxants and barbiturates. When clinicians use these regimens it is obvious that causing death is the intended outcome. Opioid drugs, however, can be titrated to relieve suffering or administered in an "overdose" with the intent to hasten death. Given the variability in the patient's condition and previous exposure to opioid drugs, scrutinizing the exact dose administered will often not be sufficient to determine whether the intent was palliative or lethal. Also, even when the clinician's intent is, in part, to hasten death, it will often not be clear whether the dose administered, in fact, contributed to causing death (Douglas et al. 2008; Sprung et al. 2008).

What ethical grounds can support an absolute prohibition on active euthanasia? Causing and intending to cause death via stopping LST is ethical to respect autonomy and relieve suffering; palliative care to relieve suffering at the risk of hastening death is also ethical. Why, then, is it necessarily unethical to administer lethal treatment in response to a patient's voluntary and informed request? For this practice is also undertaken to respect autonomy and relieve suffering. Moreover, as we argued in Chapter 1, to assume that causing death is a bad effect, which thus only can be justified in conformity with the doctrine of double effect, begs the ethical question.

Below we will take up the issue of whether the professional integrity of physicians can ground a prohibition on active euthanasia, bearing in mind that neither causation nor intention clearly distinguishes this practice from withdrawing LST and that the empirical and ethical distinction between palliative care and active euthanasia is often tenuous. Unless some credible reasons can be supplied as to why doctors *qua* doctors cannot ethically administer a lethal injection to patients under any circumstances, then it is difficult to see how these lines can be held. Before discussing this issue, we examine the distinction between refusals of LST and requests for life-ending treatment.

REFUSALS AND REQUESTS

Ethical discussion of active euthanasia compared with withdrawing LST has often been simplistic: it is presumed that either there is an absolute moral distinction between them or they are morally equivalent. Challenging the bright lines between withdrawing LST and palliative care, on the one hand, and active euthanasia, on the other, doesn't imply that there are no morally significant differences between these practices. In other words, the stance that active euthanasia can be ethically permissible in some circumstances is consistent with recognizing that it is not morally equivalent to withdrawing LST—that some moral characteristics of the latter may not characterize the former.

Although the decision to stop LST may be described as a request to clinicians to withdraw treatment, from an ethical and legal perspective it has the status of a refusal of consent for continuing treatment. Patients have a right to refuse LST. Correlatively, attending clinicians have a duty to respect this right. Medical treatment without consent violates a person's bodily integrity. Without a right to refuse treatment, patients become prisoners of medical technology. Failure to respect a person's right to refuse unwanted medical treatment is a gross interference with *personal sovereignty*, which is basic to the normative foundation of liberal democracy (Feinberg 1986, 52–97).

The idea of personal sovereignty—an inviolable zone of personal conduct and enjoyment of property free from invasion by others—has deep roots in liberal moral and political thought. In the introductory chapter to *On Liberty* Mill (1859) declared that "Over himself, over his own body and mind, the individual is sovereign" (73). Personal sovereignty involves both protective and facilitative dimensions. Recognizing personal sovereignty in the law and common mores protects individuals from unwanted intrusions on their freedom and property. It also demarcates a zone of interpersonal conduct in which individuals should have the opportunity to interact consensually with others free from external interference, provided that they do not harm third parties or violate their rights. The requirement to obtain consent protects persons from invasions by others of their personal sovereignty, thus respecting their freedom to be left alone. It also facilitates permissible interaction with others, thus respecting freedom of cooperative activity. In other words, consent and personal sovereignty go hand in hand: a zone of personal inviolability and control is manifested by respect for the ability to give and withhold consent.

The right to stop LST requires a valid refusal—that is, one that is informed and voluntary. Accordingly, to ensure that the refusal is valid, it is incumbent on clinicians to engage in careful inquiry and conversation with the patient before complying, especially because stopping treatment will lead to the patient's death. For example, a 25-year-old man injured in a motorcycle accident becomes quadriplegic and ventilator dependent. Shortly after the accident the patient requests that his ventilator be stopped so that he can die. The patient has a right to refuse treatment; however, there are good reasons for recommending that such patients take time to undergo rehabilitation and attempt to adjust to their circumstances (Patterson et al. 1993). Most of these patients find that their quality of life is satisfactory. Even though the right to refuse is clear, it is good practice to recommend that the patient hold off, both to ensure that any choice of death is voluntary and adequately informed and for the sake of promoting the person's well-being. A favorable prognosis for extended life and the irrevocability of the death-causing treatment refusal make this communicative approach desirable, especially at the early stage after the drastic injury. Yet no patient should be forced to endure unwanted treatment, and a persisting and informed decision to stop treatment by a competent patient must be respected.

A request for active euthanasia does not have the same moral status as a refusal of LST. In general, refusals and requests are not morally equivalent, although they both involve personal sovereignty (Gert et al. 1994). Valid refusals amount to authorized demands to refrain from or cease an unwanted interaction. They obligate others to comply or not to interfere. For example, A has a right to refuse a sexual advance or invitation by B, in which case B is not permitted to proceed. B may request but has no right to demand sexual intercourse with A. A is free to quit her job, and she may request to be considered for employment by another organization; however, she has no right to demand a desired job.

Medical care is somewhat more complicated. It is reasonable to see people as having a right to needed medical care and thus entitled to the help of medical professionals. Even so, patients do not have a right to receive whatever treatment they request. Whether there are *any* circumstances under which patients have a (moral) claim-right to receive a lethal injection—a right that clinicians are obliged to respect—is debatable. In any case, in declining a request for a lethal injection the physician does not violate the patient's bodily integrity. Even if an argument can be made for a right to active euthanasia under specified circumstances, it is less strongly grounded than the right to refuse treatment, and considerably more circumscribed. Incurably ill persons who find their lives intolerable retain other ways to cause their death, including stopping eating and drinking. And physicians are obligated to provide palliative care to relieve pain and other forms of physical suffering.

In assessing the distinctive moral characteristics of refusing LST and requesting active euthanasia, the moral agency of clinicians deserves attention. Consider the difference in what is being asked of clinicians in the case of these two practices. As we have noted, in withdrawing LST, the request of a competent patient to be free from an unwanted treatment, or that of an authorized surrogate on behalf of an incompetent patient, is essentially a refusal of treatment. When consent for continued treatment has been validly refused, physicians no longer have any authorization for continuing that treatment. Whether or not the attending clinician agrees with the decision to stop treatment, he or she is obligated morally and legally to comply with a valid refusal. This in no way infringes on the moral agency of the clinician, because such agency can't coherently extend to requiring patients to endure treatments that they have validly refused in a society that respects personal sovereignty. The consent that makes treatment permissible has been withdrawn.

In the case of a request for active euthanasia, a physician is being asked to intervene with a medical treatment that induces death. The physician loses moral agency if he or she is ethically required to comply with such a request from a competent patient. As a professional, the clinician must retain discretion to act in accordance with reasonable judgments about what is medically appropriate treatment. Active euthanasia could be considered medically necessary only in the most extraordinary circumstances. In almost all cases, pain and suffering can be controlled with commonly available medications in doses that fall short of directly causing the death of the patient, even if it means sedating the patient to unconsciousness (Quill et al. 2009). The rare exception might include situations in which a battlefield medic has run out of medications and has no choice but to shoot a soldier who is irreversibly dying in agony. Outside such rare circumstances, it is highly doubtful that competent medical care demands active euthanasia for any patient condition, such that it might be considered professional malpractice not to offer or provide it. It doesn't follow, however, that active euthanasia is never ethically appropriate.

A qualification is in order with respect to the distinction between requests and refusals. In ordinary life we are often confronted with requests with which we feel compelled to comply—requests that must be honored absent a strong countervailing reason to refuse. Given B's relationship with A, and the nature of A's request, B may be obligated to comply (e.g., an invitation to a family event). In some cases, a doctor–patient relationship, coupled with a shared understanding and agreement about end-of-life care, may put a physician in a position in which he or she cannot ethically refuse a request for active euthanasia.

The death of Sigmund Freud, suffering grievously from cancer of the mouth, arguably qualifies for such a case of a request for active euthanasia that obligates compliance (Miller 1991). Peter Gay, in his biography of Freud, narrates Freud's request to his long-standing personal physician and friend as follows: "Schur, you remember our 'contract' not to leave me in the lurch when the time has come. Now it is nothing but torture and makes no sense" (Gay 1988, 651). However, it is not the request in itself that carries the obligatory force. Rather, it is the relationship and shared understanding (including the physician's expressed willingness to administer lethal treatment) that obligates, making this obligation at least quasipromissory. In contrast, a valid refusal of LST by itself obligates the compliance of an attending physician who may have had only a short-term relationship with the patient and no prior agreement regarding end-of-life care.

Beauchamp and Childress sum up the distinction between refusals and requests in the context of end-of-life decisions as follows: "A health professional is obligated to honor an autonomous refusal of a life-prolonging technology, but he or she is not obligated under ordinary circumstances to honor an autonomous request for aid-in-dying [assisted suicide or active euthanasia]. However, the issue is not whether physicians are *obligated* to lend assistance in dying, but whether valid requests render it *permissible* for a physician (or some other person) to lend aid-in-dying. *Refusals* in medical settings have a moral force not found in requests, but requests do not lack all power to confer on another a right to act in response" (Beauchamp and Childress 2009, 180).

Although there is no claim-right to voluntary active euthanasia (VAE) such that physicians have a duty to comply with a suffering patient's voluntary request, might there be a liberty-right, grounded in autonomy and beneficence, to VAE from a willing physician? This would be a right of noninterference by others with a negotiated agreement. As such, it could be considered as within the zone of personal sovereignty under which individuals are free to enter into cooperative interactions with others as long as they pose no harm to third parties. However, a precondition for establishing such a (moral) right would be an argument that compliance by a willing physician is not contrary to the role morality of medicine, which we address in the next section. Additionally, to make the case that such a right should be legally recognized requires attention to policy considerations in favor of and against legalization of VAE. We take up the policy question in the final section.

ROLE MORALITY AND PROFESSIONAL INTEGRITY

Does active euthanasia violate the role morality and professional integrity of physicians? If the claim that active euthanasia lies outside the bounds of medical morality is based on it being unethical for doctors to cause death intentionally, then the argument of Chapter 1 undermines this claim. Given that doctors legitimately cause death in withdrawing LST and frequently intend to cause death, or at least cause it knowingly, what makes it intrinsically unethical for doctors to cause patients to die by giving them a lethal injection in response to a request to do so, when that request has been carefully considered by the patient in light of available alternative ways to relieve suffering?

We noted in Chapter 1 and at the beginning of this chapter, that the causal pathway to death is different in active euthanasia than in withdrawing LST. Giving the patient a lethal dose of medication induces death directly. It will kill a healthy or a sick person. Stopping a ventilator will cause death only for a patient who is incapable of adequate spontaneous respiration. (For the sake of this discussion we set aside the causal pathway in the case of stopping artificial nutrition and hydration.) Active euthanasia uses the ordinary tools of medicine—a syringe filled with drugs—to cause a patient's death. Stopping life-sustaining treatment withdraws the technological tools of medicine, resulting in a patient's death. Does this difference in the way that a patient's death is caused amount to any meaningful difference in what a physician is *permitted* to do?

To answer this question we need to examine the role morality of medicine. In general, philosophers interested in the ethics of active euthanasia have concentrated on the principles of autonomy and (general) beneficence; they have paid scant attention to whether it can be ethical for physicians to engage in this practice in view of the role morality of medicine and professional integrity, which we understand as commitment to this role morality. For example, Singer's utilitarian argument in favor of voluntary active euthanasia ignores professional morality (Singer 2003). So does Feinberg (1986) and also Dworkin (1993), approaching active euthanasia from the perspective of liberal political philosophy. Feinberg states that "[t]o the liberal, it is only the voluntariness of the death request (given its self-regarding character) that counts; pain and suffering of the life remaining are not necessary for its fulfillment" (351). Not only does this statement privilege autonomy as the governing ethical principle, it suggests that any ethical considerations relating to the professional morality of medicine are irrelevant. We submit that the professional morality of medicine is important to do justice to the full range of ethical issues relevant to active euthanasia; moreover, failure to engage this perspective ignores the deepest concerns of physicians with the legitimacy of this practice.

The role morality of medicine has often been discussed in terms of an *internal* morality. Kass, a leading critic of active euthanasia from the perspective of medicine's professional morality, describes medicine as "intrinsically a moral profession, with its own immanent principles and standards of conduct that set limits on what physicians may properly do" (Kass 1989, 28).

Although one of us (F.G.M.) has coauthored several articles explicating and endorsing a conception of the internal morality of medicine, we (now) regard the idea of professional morality being internal to the profession as problematic for several reasons. First, it is not clear whether professional morality is best characterized as internal to, or inherent in, the profession or as an application of general morality to the context of the profession. Second, the metaphor of being internal suggests, but does not strictly entail, that only members of the profession can fully appreciate the role morality proper to the profession. This tends to make professional morality insular and immune to critical evaluation by outsiders. Third, the internal morality does not encompass the whole of medical ethics or ethics as applied to medical practice, raising the question of how to distinguish the internal from the external morality (Arras 2001).

Fourth, consent generally has not been embraced as part of the internal morality of medicine, which draws its roots from the paternalistic Hippocratic tradition. Arras notes that "certain indispensable elements of contemporary medical morality, such as a duty to obtain the informed consent of patients, simply cannot be derived from an analysis of the concept or primary goals of medicine" (Arras 2001, 651). Treating consent as external to the professional role morality of medicine does not do justice to the way that it grounds the authority of medicine. To be sure, physicians possess authority that is independent of consent in the form of expertise. This includes epistemic authority, grounded in scientific knowledge, and the authority of skilled technique in performing interventional procedures. It is on account of this expertise that people seek the help of physicians. But, as a rule, physicians have no authority to intervene on behalf of patients and administer medical procedures in the absence of consent (either of the patient or an authorized surrogate). The exception of emergency medicine for incapacitated patients lacking anyone present to consent on their behalf is justified in terms of "presumed consent"—it is presumed that people want to preserve their lives and would consent to life-saving procedures if they could. Consent belongs to role morality in the context of helping professions as a basic ethical constraint, without which professionals have no authority to provide help.

Finally, the metaphor of internality suggests uniqueness of role morality to respective professions when, in fact, there is considerable overlap between various professional moralities: for example, medicine shares with law a fiduciary orientation, respect for confidentiality, concern with conflicts of interest, etc. Despite these problems, we don't reject entirely the conception of a professional role morality having an internal component. Specifically, as developed below, we see the proper goals of the profession as providing important ethical guidance and constraint on professional activities.

Kass describes medicine as "intrinsically ethical" (Kass 1989, 26). It's not clear what this means, but surely medicine is not an intrinsic good. Rather, it is instrumental to serving goals relating to health and personal well-being. Accordingly, the role morality of medicine is guided by the goals of this professional activity. In addition to being directed at specific goals, medicine should be constrained in pursuing these goals by a set of appropriate norms. Kass sees medicine as having a single *essential* goal, described as promoting health or healing. Obviously, this is central to the goals of medicine, but it is difficult to fit all the ethically legitimate activities of physicians within the orbit of promoting health or healing, even if we adopt a capacious conception of this fundamental goal. Moreover, promoting health and promoting healing are not necessarily identical. Many patients have incurable and/or progressive diseases; they need care but can't be restored to health. Additionally, given the bias of contemporary medicine toward curative and life-prolonging interventions, it is desirable to include relief of suffering as a separate goal of medicine, despite its considerable overlap with healing and promoting health.

An international group of scholars convened by the Hastings Center issued a report on the goals of medicine. It specified the following four goals: (1) "the prevention of disease and injury and the promotion and maintenance of health"; (2) "the relief of pain and suffering caused by maladies"; (3) "the care and cure of those with a malady, and the care of those who cannot be cured"; and (4) "the avoidance of premature death and the pursuit of a peaceful death" (Callahan 1996). This statement of goals of medicine is valuable for our purpose both because it is reflects an international consensus and it was developed as a general approach to defining these goals, without the specific intent of addressing the question of active euthanasia. The fourth goal is especially important for inquiry about whether active euthanasia, in some circumstances, is consistent with the professional morality of medicine. If we adopt Kass's perspective on *the* goal of medicine, understood as healing or promoting health, it is impossible for active euthanasia to be a legitimate medical practice, for in no way can this be construed under any circumstances as an intervention that promotes health or heals. This, of course, is the conclusion that Kass seeks to draw. However, it is a valid inference only if it follows from a sound conception of professional morality, including the goals of medicine. Because pursuit of a peaceful death is a valid goal of medicine—a goal that lies outside promoting health and healing—it is an open question whether active euthanasia may be in some circumstances an ethically legitimate practice in the service of this goal.

This point is bolstered by consideration of the second goal in this report— the relief of pain and suffering caused by maladies. Kass certainly includes this within his single essential goal of healing/promoting health, but because he sees relief of suffering as a part of the single goal, it necessarily excludes active euthanasia as a means to relieving suffering. Yet whether it should be excluded is the very question at issue; and this question should not be begged by defining the goals of medicine in a way that makes it impossible to include active euthanasia. In other words, given the plurality of proper goals of medicine, as aptly expressed in this report of the Hastings Center, the prohibition of active euthanasia does not follow from the meaning of the goals themselves.

In explaining the traditional Hippocratic prohibition of administering lethal medication, Kass remarks that "For the physician, at least, human life in living bodies commands respect and reverence—*by its very nature*" (38). The goals of medicine certainly entail respect for the human body, which the physician examines and treats in order to promote health. But reverence and respect for mere human biological life represents a mistaken view of medical priorities. In Chapter 3 we argue that patients diagnosed as "brain dead" remain alive. The maintenance of life in these bodies, in view of the irreversible loss of consciousness, commands respect and reverence primarily only as a source of organs to preserve life in others. Otherwise, these living bodies without a personal life are appropriately respected by stopping life support and preparing them for cremation or burial. Respect for the human body must be accompanied by respect for the person whose body it is (or was). The physician serves the patient via ministering to the body; however, in unfortunate circumstances the most appropriate service for the patient may be to help in ending bodily life. The living body commands respect and reverence primarily for the sake of the personal life that it embodies.

We contend that the goals of medicine permit VAE, to relieve suffering and pursue a peaceful death, but consideration of the full set of goals places definite constraints on the legitimacy of this practice. Clearly, VAE is in tension with promoting health, especially the commitment to preserving life that is part of this goal. As indicated above, medical practice is further constrained by a set of norms governing pursuit of these goals. In previous work, Miller and Brody endorsed the four goals of medicine described above and identified "four internal duties" incumbent on physicians: "(i) competence in the technical and humanistic skills required to practice medicine; (ii) avoiding disproportionate harms that are not balanced by the prospect of compensating medical benefits; (iii) refraining from the fraudulent misrepresentation of medicine as a scientific practice and clinical art; and (iv) fidelity to the therapeutic relationship with patients in need of care" (Miller and Brody 2001, 583). In line with our critique of the internal morality conception, we do not insist that these role morality duties should be understood as internal to medicine (as distinct from applications of general moral norms to the context of medicine). More importantly, we would add informed consent as a fundamental constraint and duty of physicians because there is no ethical foothold for medical intervention in the absence of consent.

Miller and Brody (1995) argued that none of the four duties precludes VAE as a medical intervention of last resort. Nor is there any reason to think that patients are incapable of giving informed consent to a desired lethal intervention. The second duty of proportionality of benefits and harms deserves specific attention. How can intervening to induce a patient's death be considered a benefit? Kass (1989) asserts that this is impossible: "'Better off dead' is logical nonsense... To intend and act for someone's good requires his continued existence to receive the benefit" (40). Kass is surely mistaken. Insofar as death liberates a person from intolerable and otherwise unrelievable suffering, then it is a benefit, even if this cannot be experienced. Continuing an intolerable existence can be a fate worse than death, making it reasonable to consider a person better off dead—that is, better than the alternative of continued suffering or subsisting in a state of medically induced unconsciousness while awaiting death. Furthermore, it is important not to ignore the experienced benefit to incurably ill patients of knowing that there is a swift and peaceful way out if suffering becomes unbearable.

Setting Limits

Kass observes that "The need for finding or setting limits to the use of power is especially important when the power is dangerous" (36). Callahan joins Kass in arguing that the power of medicine must be limited by excluding assisted suicide and active euthanasia: "There has been a long-standing, historical resistance to giving physicians the power to kill, precisely because of the skill they could bring to the task: if their technical power to kill were matched by a moral or legal authority to kill or assist in suicide, the way would be open for a corruption of their vocation" (Callahan 1993, 101–102).

Whether the power to kill that active euthanasia involves is so dangerous that physicians should never be permitted to wield it is an issue that we address in the next section, where we take up policy considerations. Yet, in Chapter 1 we noted that the power to sustain life in the face of life-threatening conditions, for a shorter or longer period of time, goes hand in hand with the power to cause death—to initiate the causal process that brings about death from stopping LST in conjunction with the unopposed effects of the patient's medical condition. The flipside of the technical power to stave off death is the power to cause death when those technical means are withdrawn. With the advent of LST, physicians legitimately assumed power they previously lacked, including the largely unacknowledged power to cause death when LST is stopped. Deliberately stopping LST and thus causing death has not corrupted the medical vocation. Hence it is not clear that active euthanasia, another way of causing death, inherently corrupts. Framing the issue of physician-assisted death rhetorically in terms of "killing" and "assisting in suicide" lends persuasive force to the charge of corruption; framing it in terms of "causing death" and "helping to die" leaves it open to empirical assessment as to whether such an expansion in the power of physicians (beyond stopping LST) corrupts medicine or expands its beneficence.

Limits to the power of medicine remain ethically important when the bright line is abandoned. Although the goals of medicine arguably permit active euthanasia in some circumstances, they suggest limits on the appropriate use of this life-terminating medical practice. In view of the first goal of promoting and maintaining health, physicians should never agree to a request for active euthanasia from a healthy person. To comply with such a request would grossly violate the commitments to preserve life and promote health. Not only do healthy people lack any right to assisted death on request, but it would be wrong for physicians to comply, although it would not necessarily be a wrong *to* the requesting individual.

The patient's prognosis is relevant to the legitimacy of active euthanasia. The longer a patient may live, the more a life-terminating act conflicts with the goals of promoting health and avoiding a premature death. Limitation of active euthanasia to the terminally ill, however, would be arbitrary. If patients are suffering intolerably with no hope for relief, then a longer prognosis of continued suffering makes them worse off than those who are terminally ill. To be eligible for VAE, patients should be incurably ill. Furthermore, in view of the resources of palliative care, VAE should be a last resort treatment, when the patient's persisting suffering cannot be relieved adequately by standard medical means. To be sure, sedation to unconsciousness is always possible; but, absent appeal to the sanctity of human biological life, it is hard to see a sedated existence pending death as preferable to a chosen death by active euthanasia for those who find their lives intolerable in the face of incurable illness. Incurably ill patients who request help in ending their lives before they reach a state of intolerable suffering pose a greater challenge to professional integrity. For these patients, a clinician's pledge not to abandon the patient, coupled with an agreement to be available to consider this intervention when suffering becomes intolerable, may help to maintain (relative) health and serve to adequately relieve anticipatory distress.

Is active euthanasia ethically acceptable only in response to the current voluntary request of a competent patient? We are not convinced that nonvoluntary active euthanasia is never justified. However, we suggest that, as a rule, there is a strong burden of proof against it, especially in view of alternative means of palliative care to relieve suffering. One circumstance in which nonvoluntary active euthanasia appears justifiable in principle is when surrogate decision makers choose to stop artificial nutrition and hydration, as in the case of

Nancy Cruzan. If the decision to stop treatment knowing that death will occur is justifiable, what could be wrong with a physician giving the patient a lethal injection instead of waiting several days for death to occur by dehydration?

Specifying the scope and limits of permissible VAE is inherently difficult. Perhaps the most compelling cases are those of patients near death who are suffering intensely and want to end their lives: for example, a patient with advanced metastatic cancer who is experiencing severe pain and/or shortness of breath and does not want to live out her remaining days in a sedated state. The justification for a planned death with physician assistance in this circumstance is bolstered when close family members or intimate partners responsible for the care of the patient concur. Also compelling is the case of a patient with an advanced progressive disease such as amyotrophic lateral sclerosis (ALS) with a known downward course who chooses not to endure the end stage, including ventilator dependence.

How about elderly patients with multiple health problems and progressive functional decline who no longer wish to continue living? David Eddy wrote a moving narrative of his mother's death by forgoing food and water (Eddy 1994). Mrs. Eddy, at age 84 years, became bedridden, incontinent, subject to deteriorating eyesight, and confined to a nursing home after experiencing a cascade of acute medical problems. She was not dying but had irreversibly lost her capacity for independent living—a loss that mattered greatly to her. Having felt that she had lived a full life, she decided to seek death because of what she regarded as a drastic and permanent deterioration in her quality of life. In conversation with her physician son, she considered but rejected clandestine assisted suicide by ingesting lethal medication. After surviving a bout of pneumonia, despite refusing antibiotics, she chose to stop eating and drinking. Her physician agreed to help keep her comfortable while she awaited death, which arrived several days later. Suppose instead that she had requested her physician to give her a lethal injection and he concurred with her plan. (We set aside any concerns about legal liability.) What would be wrong with the physician assisting her death in this case?

Compare Mrs. Eddy's situation with the case of Edward Brongersma, an 86-year-old Dutch man who requested euthanasia owing to "life fatigue" (Huxtable and Moller 2007). According to his physician, who complied with the request, Brongersma "experienced life as futile, was unhappy and lonely." The physician was prosecuted and found guilty of not following the established Dutch guidelines for euthanasia but was not punished because he acted in good faith. Huxtable and Moller argue that the principles of respect for autonomy and patient-centered beneficence support VAE for Brongersma. (They note some "practical" reasons against VAE in this sort of case.) Yet multiple reasons of professional integrity make VAE out of bounds in this case.

Though suffering from existential distress, the patient appeared to have no diagnosable malady. If the patient was depressed, antidepressant medication and/or psychotherapy, rather than assisted death would be an appropriate response. Moreover, in view of potentially effective psychosocial intervention, it is difficult to see how in this case VAE could ever be an appropriate option of last resort. The patient might autonomously refuse such nonmedical help, but this doesn't make it acceptable for a physician to comply with a request for lethal treatment. Although the patient was old, he was not functionally disabled, in contrast to Mrs. Eddy. His situation lacks any grave compromise to health, making physician assistance in death contrary to professional role morality.

A more challenging case from the perspective of professional integrity might be the situation of a quadriplegic person who has lived for a considerable period of time after a devastating injury but now no longer wishes to continue living. If he were ventilator dependent, then he would have a right to die by choosing to stop treatment. But suppose he is not. He is incapable of killing himself other than by refusing to eat and drink. Assuming that it would be ethically acceptable for him to die in this manner, would there be anything wrong with a physician performing VAE after careful consideration of the request? The fact that the physician would be causing the patient's death is not ethically decisive, as physicians also cause death when stopping a ventilator. The quantity of life that is given up merits consideration, but so does the quality of life as perceived by the patient. In any case, it is far from obvious why it is considered fully justifiable for clinicians to cause the death of a ventilator-dependent quadriplegic who refuses continued mechanical ventilation but not ethically justifiable to provide a lethal injection for a patient in the same situation with the exception of not needing a ventilator to breathe. Although the distinction between requests and refusals, discussed above, is relevant to this pair of cases, it doesn't follow that it would be unethical for a physician to perform VAE at the request of this patient who lacks the opportunity to die by stopping LST.

Patients with dementia who seek death pose difficult issues. Janet Adkins chose to die by assisted suicide, arranged by Jack Kevorkian, when she was in the early stage of Alzheimer's disease and still at a high level of functioning (Betzold 1993, 41–82). Such a death seems premature and physician assistance ethically problematic, if not unethical. Suppose, however, that someone makes a clear advance directive stating that she wants active euthanasia if she becomes so demented that she is no longer able to recognize her family or interact in a meaningful way with others. Might active euthanasia be justifiable in such a case?

It is not our intent to develop a comprehensive casuistry for the ethical legitimacy of VAE. We reiterate two key points. First, active euthanasia as a last resort in response to intolerable and refractory suffering from incurable illness is not inherently contrary to the role morality of medicine. Second, this role morality, consisting of goals of medicine and ethical constraints on the pursuit of these goals, limits the scope of legitimate active euthanasia. Above we stressed that physicians are moral agents. Although they are obliged to honor death-causing refusals of treatment, as there is no authorization for continued treatment that has been refused, they are not obliged to comply with requests for assisted suicide or active euthanasia. The role morality of medicine gives substantive guidance to physicians who are prepared to provide lethal treatment in response to valid requests. It imposes some general constraints on the scope of acceptable active euthanasia, though necessarily leaving room for discretionary and responsible judgment. Because they are moral agents, physicians should be free to refuse any and all requests for active euthanasia, with the exception of promises to provide this help in the future under agreed on conditions.

Given that VAE is necessarily in some tension with the goals of medicine, individual physicians are entitled to adopt a policy of refusing to perform this last resort practice, just as they are free to refuse to perform abortion if it violates their conscience. Indeed, conscientious refusal is on stronger grounds with respect to VAE. Patients seeking death by active euthanasia can request other physicians to help. Moreover, suffering can almost always be controlled by means that fall short of causing death; and patients are always free to kill themselves by stopping eating and drinking. In contrast, women seeking abortion have no acceptable recourse when physicians refuse to help them.

Understanding VAE as a treatment of last resort is critical to its compatibility with medical morality. VAE is not appropriate if there are interventions that can adequately relieve suffering short of causing death. What makes the suffering patient's situation unbearable will depend first and foremost on the patient's judgment in light of the consideration of available alternatives. However, it remains up to the physician who receives a request for VAE to decide whether to concur. Alternative palliative care interventions are preferable, other things being equal, to VAE because the patient may find continued living with supportive care worthwhile; and they are preferable if they meet the needs of the patient because clinicians can thereby avoid lethal treatment. VAE should never be a "quick fix."

Despite the existence of a range of cases of VAE that appear ethically compelling, the fact that there are alternatives to active euthanasia might suggest that there is no need for physicians to adopt this practice, even when limited to a last resort option. Yet if voluntary active euthanasia as a last resort is compatible with medical role morality, as we have argued, why should patients be denied the opportunity to choose a swift, peaceful, and dignified death from physicians willing to provide this help, as an alternative to a slow death from dehydration following forgoing food and water (lasting up to 2 weeks or more), with or without sedation to unconsciousness?

It is important to recognize the limits of our argument that VAE is compatible with the role morality of physicians. We do not claim that it is *required* by professional ethics. Physicians who fail to provide adequate palliative care in response to the suffering of patients fail to fulfill their role obligations; this constitutes incompetent medical practice. In contrast, physicians who refuse to perform VAE do not contravene their role obligations to patients. In other words, we see VAE as a permissible but not obligatory component of patient care. But if patients have a right to receive palliative care, shouldn't they also have a right to active euthanasia on request when, from the perspective of the patient, ending life is the only way to relieve their suffering?

Medical treatment to relieve suffering while not deliberately ending life is one thing; relieving suffering *by* deliberately ending life is another. The latter arguably lies outside the scope of palliative care, as there are few situations in which lethal treatment is necessary to relieve suffering. Patients have a right to medically indicated treatment, not to any treatment that they demand. Likewise, there are no situations in which strictly cosmetic surgery is medically necessary. Just as cosmetic surgery is permissible but falls outside the scope of a right to medical care (and thus typically is not funded by health plans), so VAE falls outside the scope of palliative care to which patients have a claim-right. Failure to provide adequate palliative care, from an ethical perspective, abandons suffering patients in need of help. However, in view of the power of competent palliative care to relieve suffering, including sedation to unconsciousness as a last resort, patients are not abandoned to intolerable suffering when individual clinicians, as well as the medical community, refuse to comply with requests for active euthanasia. The grounds for a claim-right to active euthanasia—a right that clinicians are duty-bound to respect—are not clear. The professional status of physicians includes the authority, within the scope of established professional standards, to determine whether a medical intervention is appropriate. If patients had the right to demand life-terminating treatment, then it would override the professional autonomy of physicians. The claim of professional autonomy is especially strong in this context, as the requested intervention is to induce death by administering lethal treatment.

Even in the Netherlands, active euthanasia is seen as a matter of the physician's discretion, to be used as an option of last resort in accordance with the clinical judgment that there are no reasonable alternatives. There is a good reason for this: VAE can't be limited to a measure of last resort, consistent with professional integrity, unless physicians are free to refuse requests from patients who are not seen as appropriate candidates for lethal treatment. Otherwise, this practice becomes solely a matter of patient autonomy, constrained only by the assessment of whether the request is voluntary and informed. Clinicians are obligated to comply with valid refusals of treatment and provide palliative care to relieve suffering. Although voluntary active euthanasia may be ethically permissible, clinicians are not obligated to comply with patient requests.

Disability and Medical Authority

As a transition to addressing policy considerations, an objection to physician-assisted death with respect to its allegedly deleterious social implications merits attention (Bickenbach 1998). Medical intervention to end the lives of incurably ill or disabled individuals lends the authority of medicine to the view that these people, and others like them, have lives that are not worth living. As such, it devalues the existence of classes of vulnerable people and thus reinforces prejudicial social attitudes relating to the quality of life of persons with disability. This not only injures their sense of self-worth and worth in the eyes of others, it may put pressure on them to consider their lives unworthy and thus to request VAE.

In principle, this objection also applies to withdrawing LST, especially for those who are not imminently dying. Concerns about devaluing the lives of the disabled and the voluntariness of their decisions to withdraw treatment warrant careful evaluation of treatment refusals; however, it would be unfairly discriminatory to deny or limit the right of disabled patients to stop LST. Why, then, should it count as a decisive objection against VAE? Nevertheless, the force of this objection is stronger in the case of VAE. Clinicians are obligated to comply with valid refusals, which withdraw authorization for continued treatment. Accordingly, compliance does not count as an endorsement of patients' judgments that their lives are not worth living. In VAE, however, physicians have discretion as to whether to comply with requests for assisted death, making them more implicated in judgments about the patients' quality of life.

On closer scrutiny, this objection fails to hold up. Physicians who agree to requests for VAE are committed to providing help that is desired by suffering patients. To make this help ethically acceptable, they need to assess the decision-making capacity of the patient and the severity of suffering, to discuss alternative means of relieving it that allow the patient to live, and to judge that VAE qualifies as a last resort. Although they are unlikely to comply unless they see the request as reasonable given the patient's condition and values, their compliance logically entails no judgment about the class of patients with the same medical condition. VAE is a form of personalized care, provided by individual physicians at their discretion; it does not involve any collective, authoritative stance on what types of lives are not worth living.

The same objection has been lodged against abortion. For example, critics argue that the common practice of aborting fetuses diagnosed with Down's syndrome devalues the lives of individuals with this condition. But this is a non sequitur. The practice of abortion in no way entails that the lives of persons with mental retardation are not worth living. Individuals with Down's syndrome have an equal right to live and deserve to be valued as human beings. The logical critique, however, doesn't necessarily extinguish the psychological force of this objection. Thus, it is incumbent on advocates of VAE to make clear that their stance has nothing to do with devaluing the lives of the disabled and incurably ill. VAE is not a socially preferred option for any conditions but a matter of individual choice and negotiation with willing physicians. The point discussed above that active euthanasia is almost never medically necessary is relevant in this regard. If there were medical conditions that warranted lethal treatment, then this would lend the social authority of medicine to the view that certain lives are not worth living.

VAE differs radically from the Nazi "euthanasia" program, under which thousands of mentally ill and neurologically disabled individuals were killed in gas chambers (Friedlander 1995). This program operated under a state-supported ideology of "racial hygiene," embraced by the medical establishment, which was deployed to judge classes of people as having lives "unworthy of life" (Proctor 1988). There was nothing voluntary about the life-ending interventions on these institutionalized patients; nor was it directed to the relief of suffering. Although it is a mistake to see VAE as having anything to do with the Nazi extermination policies, which are misleadingly described as "euthanasia," the potential for abuse and the slide down the slippery slope must be addressed.

POLICY CONSIDERATIONS

The upshot of our analysis so far is that there are no grounds for drawing an ethical bright line permitting withdrawing LST and palliative care but prohibiting active euthanasia. Neither appeal to causation and intention, on the one hand, nor the role morality of medicine, on the other, supports an ethical prohibition of active euthanasia. It doesn't follow that a practice of VAE, even if circumscribed as suggested above, should be legalized in the United States, as it is in the Netherlands and Belgium. Three major reasons posed against a policy of legalization are that it would undermine trust in physicians, that there is insufficient need for this practice in view of legally available alternatives, and that legalization would promote intolerable abuses.

Trust

Gaylin, Kass, Pelegrino, and Siegler, in their statement on active euthanasia described above, declared, "This issue touches medicine at its very moral center, if this moral center collapses, if physicians become killers or are even merely licensed to kill, the profession—and therewith, each physician—will never again be worthy of trust and respect as healer and comforter and protector of life in all its frailty" (Gaylin et al. 1988). The authors are surely right that the integrity of medicine as a profession depends on trust. Vulnerability to the consequences of disease or injury and the prospect of death prompts persons to become patients by seeking the care of physicians. Trust makes it possible psychologically and morally to assume the patient role, which involves permitting doctors, who may be strangers, to probe our bodies and submitting to the risks and burdens of invasive procedures. Whereas our vulnerability as embodied persons gives rise to the need for trust in physicians, this very trust makes patients vulnerable. As Annette Baier observes, "Trust is accepted vulnerability to another's power to harm one, a power inseparable from the power to look after some aspect of one's good" (Baier 1994, 153).

Stanley Reiser aptly describes medicine as "this remarkable social institution whose members must daily prove themselves worthy of a crucial trust: that they will never take advantage of the vulnerability that is the hallmark of the patients who appear before them" (Reiser 1993, 130). Patients trust their physicians to use their skills to help, rather than to harm; for in withholding, withdrawing, or administering medical interventions, physicians have the power to produce the ultimate harm of wrongful death. The vulnerability of patients and the power of physicians must not be abused by acts or omissions that unjustly take (or risk) the lives of patients. As indicated in the quote from Gaylin and colleagues above, opponents of active euthanasia commonly argue that institutionalizing and legitimating this practice would undermine trust by patients and society at large. How can persons trust doctors who have the socially sanctioned power to kill patients? If physicians possessed the *unilateral* authority to decide when patients "need" active euthanasia, then trust would be undermined. But this sort of authority is contrary to personal sovereignty and the ethical constraint of consent. If the practice of active euthanasia is limited to competent patients who voluntarily request help in terminating their lives and who are adequately informed about available options of treatment and palliative care, VAE does not constitute an abuse of trust.

To be sure, suffering patients facing progressive disability, terminal illness, or continued diminished quality of life and dependence on others are highly vulnerable. They are liable to distorted thinking, fear of pain and humiliation, and depressed mood. As a result, their capacity for autonomous decision making may be impaired. In addition, dependent patients may feel pressured to end their lives to avoid burdening others. A request for active euthanasia should be regarded by clinicians as the occasion for inquiry, conversation, and negotiation, not the signal for immediate lethal intervention. (The same holds for a request to stop LST.) Sensitive and thorough discussion of the patient's situation and options for treatment and supportive care can help discriminate between rational and irrational decisions to terminate life. Being vulnerable, such patients need protection and care. But they also need respect for their considered judgments regarding how to live and to die.

Patients who resolve to end their lives after due consideration and discussion waive their right not to be killed. When the decision is voluntary and informed, the physician acts as the agent of the patient, not as the arbiter of death. The patient's voluntary request and informed authorization are a precondition for making active euthanasia, from the patient's perspective a benefit, and not a harm. In the practice of VAE, doctors kill patients, but they don't take their lives from them, as in criminal homicide. Hence, we conclude that there is no intrinsic compromising of trust associated with the practice of voluntary active euthanasia. Whether this practice, in fact, reduces the trust of patients in their physicians is an empirical question. Public opinion surveys in the United States indicate that only a relatively small minority of the public believes that trust would be undermined by legalizing PAS and voluntary active euthanasia (van der Maas and Emanuel 1998, 168; Hall et al. 2005). The practice of euthanasia has strong support from the public in the Netherlands, suggesting that it has not adversely affected trust in the medical profession (van der Maas et al. 1995).

Although VAE is not legal in any jurisdiction of the United States, Oregon and Washington have a growing experience with legalized PAS, which has been practiced in Oregon since 1997. Although we are not aware of any studies that directly address the effect that this legislation and practice have had on trust of society in the medical profession, reviews have generally suggested that the practice has been limited and relatively noncontroversial (Okie 2005). In the absence of more direct data, however, we can only speculate about the probable impact on trust of introducing a legal practice of voluntary active euthanasia in the United States.

Benefits

What is extent of the need for VAE? As discussed above, from a strictly medical perspective, it is questionable whether any patients need active euthanasia in view of palliative care alternatives, including sedation to unconsciousness. Although medical criteria are relevant to the ethics of VAE, including the legitimacy of physician involvement, it is not a medical issue as to whether this procedure of last resort is ethically appropriate for the situation of a given patient, all things considered. Rather, in light of reasonable eligibility criteria, which should reflect professional integrity constraints, and appropriate regulatory guidelines and procedures, it is a matter to be negotiated between physicians and patients after careful deliberation.

How many patients are likely to be helped by ethically appropriate VAE? Estimates are necessarily speculative. Emanuel (1999) examined available empirical data from the United States and arrived at an estimate of 25,000 or fewer dying Americans each year. His estimate is open to question, however, because it focused only on terminally ill patients suffering from unremitting pain. Unremitting pain is rarely the primary reason for requesting active euthanasia (van der Maas and Emanuel 1998, 155). Moreover, VAE arguably should not be limited to terminally ill patients but should also include those who are incurably ill and have unrelievable suffering.

Another way to arrive at an estimate of need or benefit is to apply the Dutch data on the incidence of VAE and assisted suicide to the United States. (Assisted suicide is much less prevalent in the Netherlands, and for the sake of this estimate we combine the numbers of those receiving VAE and PAS.) Four extensive epidemiological surveys in the Netherlands (1990, 1995, 2001, and 2005) indicate the following percentages of all deaths that are due to VAE and PAS: 1.9%, 2.6%, 2.8%, and 1.8%, respectively (Rietjens et al. 2009). Averaging over the four study periods yields a mean of 2.3% of all deaths. (PAS averaged only 0.2% over this period.) Applied to the 2.4 million annual deaths in the United States, this would suggest a total "needing" VAE of 55,200 patients per year. It is dubious to assume that all the cases of VAE and PAS in the Netherlands were ethically appropriate. To be conservative, we might assume that only half of these physician-assisted deaths were ethically appropriate. This would yield an estimate of at least 27,600 patients per year who would be appropriate for VAE in the United States, somewhat higher than Emanuel's estimate.

This estimate represents a large number of people who could benefit from VAE, though only a small percentage of annual deaths. If nothing else, these speculative estimates suggest that it would be false to conclude that there is no need for the practice. Whether the benefits justify the risks of harmful social consequences, especially terminating the lives of some patients inappropriately, is the key policy question.

Abuse

In theory, the potential for abuse is much greater in the case of active euthanasia than withdrawing LST. Anyone can be killed by a lethal injection, whereas withdrawing treatment can cause the death only of those who are receiving life support and are unable to live without it. What counts as abuse of active euthanasia is a matter of controversy; however, concern has focused primarily on nonvoluntary euthanasia—intentional life-terminating interventions of patients without their explicit request and informed consent. Critics argue that legalizing VAE will inevitably lead to active euthanasia of patients who are mentally incapacitated or who request active euthanasia under the influence of depression, financial worries, concerns about being a burden on others, or suffering that could be relieved by standard palliative care (Emanuel 1999; Arras 1998).

Much of the debate over abuses associated with active euthanasia has focused on the Netherlands, in view of its long-standing practice and a relative abundance of empirical research. After a nearly 20-year period of tolerating VAE by declining to prosecute doctors who followed official guidelines, the Dutch legalized this practice in 2002. As summarized by Rietjens and colleagues, euthanasia performed by physicians is legal under the following six conditions: "1. The patient's request is voluntary and well-considered; 2. The patient's suffering is unbearable and hopeless; 3. The patient is informed about his situation and prospects; 4. There are no reasonable alternatives; 5. Another independent physician should be consulted; and 6. The termination of life should be performed with due medical care and attention" (Rietjens et al. 2009, 273–274). Noteworthy about these guidelines is that only VAE is legal, there is no requirement of terminal illness, and the practice is justifiable only as a last resort in response to otherwise unrelievable suffering.

Despite these guidelines, which prevailed prior to formal legalization, surveys of physicians conducted from 1990 to 2005 indicate a continuing small-scale practice of what appears to be nonvoluntary active euthanasia. The percentage of all deaths from "ending of life without an explicit request" is estimated as 0.8% in 1990, 0.7% in 1995, 0.7% in 2001, and 0.4% in 2005 (Rietjens et al. 2009). As compared with the practice of VAE, active euthanasia without request predominantly involves older patients, more often occurs in the hospital rather than at home, and the drugs used are mostly opioids, in contrast to the recommended regimen for legal euthanasia of neuromuscular relaxants and/or barbiturates (Rietjens et al. 2007). According to the results of physician surveys, in approximately half of these cases the physician acted in response to prior wishes of the patient but without an explicit request; in the other half, the patients were fully incompetent and physicians had no information about their wishes. In all cases, physicians reported consulting with family members. Physicians estimated that their intervention shortened the patient's life by 1 week or less in 80% of the cases.

Rietjens and colleagues, in a systematic survey of data relating to life-terminating acts without an explicit request, suggest that these cases closely resemble those in which physicians report administering drugs to alleviate symptoms with the risk of hastening death but without an explicit (primary) intention to do so (Rietjens et al. 2007). Given the ambiguity of intentions and the lack of clarity about exactly what acts qualify as active euthanasia, it is difficult to determine how to classify these cases. On the one hand, they may be no different than standard palliative care for suffering patients close to death. On the other hand, they may be seen as nonvoluntary euthanasia. Indeed, it is possible that many of the cases classified as alleviating symptoms might also be seen as nonvoluntary euthanasia. Is the intention to hasten death ethically significant when physicians administer opioids in response to the suffering of patients who are imminently dying? Whether this reported practice of seemingly nonvoluntary euthanasia represents abuse is debatable. Judgment is difficult in the absence of a detailed examination of particular cases. Whatever we think about this practice from an ethical perspective, the data suggest that it has not increased over time.

Considerable controversy has developed over the Dutch practice of active euthanasia of severely impaired newborns (Chervenak and McCullough 2006; Lindemann and Verkerk 2008). Although contrary to the law, an institutional policy has been established under which physicians are not prosecuted if they follow specified guidelines. We do not discuss this practice, in view of the contextual details that need to be addressed to assess whether it might be ethically justified. In any case, there is no question that this practice represents nonvoluntary active euthanasia.

The potential for abuse from legalizing active euthanasia should not be assessed in a vacuum. It is important also to consider the potential for abuse that comes from the covert practice of active euthanasia despite its being illegal. Legalization has the advantage of permitting formal regulation. Explicit guidelines, mandatory consultation with other clinicians, and required reporting provide greater assurance that active euthanasia is limited to ethically appropriate interventions of last resort in response to severe suffering and voluntary requests (Miller et al. 1994). However, no workable regulatory policy would be fail-safe. Moreover, it is reasonable to anticipate that legalization would substantially expand the practice of active euthanasia and thus give rise to a greater *potential* for abuse. On the other hand, the potential for abuse of vulnerable patients is also considerable in the case of withdrawing LST, especially for incompetent patients. With the rare exception of disputed cases reviewed by the courts, decisions to withdraw life support are made without standard procedures to assess the decisions of patients and surrogate decision makers and without formal oversight. Hence, there is no way to know the extent of abuse that our society has been prepared to tolerate in recognizing the right to refuse life-sustaining treatment. The fact that withdrawal of LST occurs for the most part in health care institutions provides a level of informal oversight by a team of responsible clinicians and caregivers. Active euthanasia is much more likely to occur in patients' homes. But if these patients are enrolled in a hospice, then a care-giving team is also involved. It is an empirical issue, on which there is little evidence, as to whether expanding the scope of legitimate, legally permissible death-causing acts by clinicians to include VAE would foster intolerable abuses, which could not be obviated by reasonable regulatory procedures.

As argued above, we see no convincing reasons why VAE should be considered unethical for physicians. But this leaves open the ethics of institutionalizing or legalizing this practice. If individuals had a claim-right to VAE, on a par with the right to refuse treatment, then legalization would be ethically necessary, regardless of the potential for abuse. Arguably, a weaker liberty-right to negotiate VAE with a willing physician can be grounded in personal sovereignty. This suggests that the burden of proof should fall on critics who oppose legalization, especially when accompanied by a regulatory scheme that aims to ensure that physician-administered lethal treatment is limited to a last resort by patients who make voluntary, informed decisions. Nevertheless, reasonable people certainly will differ over whether the potential for abuse warrants refraining from legalization. Our aim is not to reach a verdict on this controversial policy question, but rather to examine the ethical issues relevant to answering it. If we believe that the practice of active euthanasia in the Netherlands is justified, it doesn't follow that it would also be justifiable to legalize VAE in the United States. The Netherlands has universal health coverage, a well-developed system of primary care (with typically long-term relationships between doctor and patient), and a comprehensive government-sponsored social safety net. Because all of these are currently lacking in the United States, there is greater reason to be concerned about abuse of vulnerable patients, which may outweigh the cost to liberty from continuing to prohibit VAE (and assisted suicide).

SUMMING UP

In this chapter and in the previous chapter we have discussed several ways in which patients end their lives in contemporary medicine: (1) withholding of treatment such as antibiotics or mechanical ventilation, (2) withdrawing LST, (3) refusing to eat and drink, (4) receiving pain medication to relieve suffering that hastens death, (5) self-administering prescribed lethal treatment, and (6) physician-administered lethal treatment. These practices differ with respect to causation of death (when death is caused), clinician intent, and the certainty that death will ensue. Physicians may stand by and merely allow the patient to die in (1) and (3); they may cause, or contribute to causing, death in (2), (4), and (5); and they induce death in (6). Physician intentions are apt to be more or less ambiguous across the spectrum, though in some of these ways of dying clinicians clearly intend to cause death. Physician intervention is certain to be the *sole* cause of death only in (6).

Despite these differences, we have seen no grounds for drawing any bright lines along this spectrum of end-of-life practices, such that some of them are morally permitted and others are strictly forbidden. The core values of patient autonomy and well-being support each of these practices, given appropriate justificatory conditions, including, but not limited to, authorization from the patient or surrogate deciding on the patient's behalf. None of these practices is categorically incompatible with the role morality of medicine, though it places limits on assisted suicide and active euthanasia; among other considerations, they are justifiable only as measures of last resort.

It doesn't follow that these practices are morally indistinguishable. Patients have claim-rights to refuse treatment and to receive palliative care that risks hastening death; accordingly, physicians are obligated to honor these refusals, when valid, and provide needed palliative care, even to the point of sedation to unconsciousness. In contrast, from an ethical perspective, patients have no right to receive lethal treatment on demand and physicians have discretion as to whether to honor these requests. It is arguable, however, that personal sovereignty should be seen as including a liberty-right to negotiate assisted death with a willing physician. Nevertheless, owing to the potential for abuse, it remains an open question as to whether physician-assisted death, by prescribing or administering lethal treatment, should be a legal option (subject to appropriate regulatory safeguards).

These practices do not exhaust the ways in which physicians may legitimately cause the death of patients in contemporary medicine. Largely unacknowledged is causing death in the context of vital organ donation. We turn to this in subsequent chapters, beginning with an examination of changes in the standards for determining death in the era of intensive care medicine and organ transplantation.

3

Death and the Brain

For most of human history, the determination of death has been clear and non-controversial. Death was diagnosed when a person was cold, blue, and stiff. But over just a few decades in the latter part of the twentieth century, coinciding with the development of intensive care medicine and organ transplantation, a radically different understanding of death was introduced and took hold, the view that death could be determined entirely in terms of the functions of the human brain. This view became rapidly and widely accepted around the world, albeit with some notable qualifications and pockets of exceptions (Capron 2001; Wijdicks 2002). In this chapter we undertake a critical examination of determining death on the basis of brain functioning, focusing mainly on the established position that regards death of the entire brain as constituting death of the human being. Whereas "brain death" has been explained as constituting death on the basis of a biological definition of death, we argue that this is mistaken in view of the extensive biological functioning maintained by individuals diagnosed as brain dead. Additionally, in Chapter 4 we contend that the rival definition of death based on the concept of a person and the function of consciousness is deficient both conceptually and practically. Although a biological conception of death in terms of the irreversible functioning of the organism as a whole is most appropriate for medicine and public policy, our current practices of organ transplantation are incompatible with this biological definition. These practices rely on brain death to make transplantation of vital organs compatible with the *dead donor rule*, which stipulates that donors must be dead prior to organ procurement. We argue, however, that individuals diagnosed correctly in accordance with the criteria of "brain death" remain (biologically) alive. Accordingly, we maintain that an ethical reconstruction of vital organ donation is required, which justifies procuring vital organs from still-living patients. This is the topic we take up in Chapter 6.

HISTORICAL CONSIDERATIONS

Most of those who live in modern Western civilizations, when asked where their "essence" resides, will refer to a place an inch or two behind the center of their eyes. Not surprisingly, the concept of brain death first emerged and has been most readily accepted in the West. As Hans-Martin Sass has observed, brain death is consonant with the humanistic Greco-Roman as well as the religious Judeo-Christian perspectives that differentiate between the mortal body and the immortal soul and interpret the ontological "nature" of humans in terms of "the *differentia specifica* of reasoning, communicating and self-communicating" (Sass 1992). This Cartesian dualism, along with identification of the soul with the mind, has quite naturally led to the conclusion that the functioning of the brain, as the physical substrate for mental processes, is a necessary condition for continued residence of the soul within the body. Indeed, the concept of brain death has met with little resistance among most proponents of Christian theology.

Even in the West, however, questions about whether death should be defined in terms of the vital functions of circulation and respiration rather than the neurological functions of the brain were largely theoretical prior to the development of mechanical ventilation. For most of history, the transition from life to death was swift, as reflected in the phrase, "the moment of death." Regardless of the cause, both the vital functions and the neurological functions tended to cease nearly simultaneously, making uncertainty about the "true" definition of death of little practical importance. An exception to this was death that followed decapitation. During the French Revolution, for example, a Parisian pathologist examining victims of the guillotine wondered about these questions when he wrote, "One hour after the execution the heart still beats; yet this man's existence was over, he had lost his personality, and yet his heart was beating" (Pope Pius XII 1957a, 393, 396). But aside from intellectual curiosities such as these, there were no practical reasons to seek greater precision or clarity in the determination of death.

With the developments in the use of mechanical ventilation that occurred following World War II, however, all of this changed. Suddenly these questions about the nature of death became both clinically and philosophically relevant. Because the neural pacemaker for diaphragmatic contraction and thereby spontaneous respiration resides in the brainstem, patients with severe injury to this portion of the brain stop breathing and quickly manifest all of the typical signs of death. After the development of mechanical ventilation, however, this function of the brainstem could be replaced by an external mechanism for sustaining respiration. With the continuation of respiration, all of the body's other vital processes also continue to function, including spontaneous heartbeat and circulation, digestion and excretion, and growth and healing.

A paper published by French neurophysiologists in 1959 is often credited as the first to explore some of the conceptual implications of this use of mechanical ventilation. They coined the term "coma depasse" (beyond coma) to describe the state of patients with devastating brain injury who were kept alive with mechanical ventilation (Mollaret and Goulon 1959). Whereas those who went to the guillotine underwent anatomical decapitation, the patients described by these scientists were considered to have suffered physiological decapitation. (We challenge this equation of brain death with physiological decapitation below.)

Speculation about using neurological criteria to diagnose death remained mostly matters for academic debate, however, until developments in another field of medicine, that of organ transplantation, suddenly made this topic very urgent. In 1967, Christian Barnard performed the first heart transplant in Cape Town, initiating a new era in the capacity for medicine to rescue patients from life-threatening organ failure (Barnard 1967, 1987). Although the donor in this case had clearly suffered severe brain damage, the event raised unanswered questions, such as whether the donor was dead at the time the heart was removed for transplantation, and if not, then whether the physicians killed the donor by removing his heart.

The following year, in 1968, Harvard anesthesiologist Henry Beecher headed an ad hoc committee at Harvard Medical School to address these issues. Although their report acknowledged that the committee's deliberations were driven in part by the development of organ transplantation, they also observed that without further legal and ethical clarification about the status of severely brain-injured patients, physicians were prohibited from withdrawing mechanical ventilation, since doing so would cause the death of these patients, in violation of ethical and legal standards. As a consequence, they argued, physicians would be forced to continue treatment on patients who had no hope of recovery, causing suffering for their family members and a scarcity of intensive care beds for other patients in need (Ad Hoc Committee 1968).

In retrospect, we can find hints that Beecher and his colleagues knew that they were making a conceptual leap in equating severe neurological injury with death. For example, the title of their seminal paper was "A Definition of Irreversible Coma, Report of the Ad Hoc Committee of the Harvard Medical School to Examine the Definition of Brain Death." The title suggests that although they were confident in claiming a criterion for defining irreversible coma, they were only implying (without argument) that this might also be a criterion for determining death. A parallel process also occurred in the United Kingdom, where in 1976 a medical committee stated that "permanent functional death of the brainstem constitutes brain death and that once this has occurred further artificial support is fruitless and should be withdrawn," clearly asserting that brain death was a criterion for justifying the withdrawal of life support, while being ambivalent about whether it was a criterion for declaring death (Medical Royal Colleges and their Faculties in the United Kingdom 1976). On both sides of the Atlantic, the concept of brain death was developed in terms of other concepts (irreversible coma or the justified withdrawal of life support) without ever providing any clear argument or justification for why the criteria for diagnosing "brain death" coincide with death of the human being.

With the rapid development of organ transplantation around the world, the pressure to define the ethical and legal status of potential organ donors became more pressing. Kansas became the first state to adopt a version of the Harvard criteria into statutory law in 1970. This law permitted surgeons to declare potential organ donors dead on the basis of neurological criteria prior to the removal of vital organs, thereby relieving concerns about whether the physicians were killing the patients during the organ procurement procedure (President's Commission 1981, 127). The situation remained ambiguous throughout the 1970s, however, with the halting and patchwork adoption of brain death criteria by individual states.

In an attempt to create a unified approach to the problem, in 1980 a President's Commission was charged with developing a model definition of death that could be recommended to the states. This resulted in the Uniform Determination of Death Act (UDDA), which states that "An individual who has sustained either (1) irreversible cessation of circulatory or respiratory functions, or (2) irreversible cessation of all functions of the entire brain, including the brainstem, is dead. A determination of death must be made in accordance with accepted medical standards" (President's Commission 1981, 2).

The UDDA, or similar legislation with only minor modifications, is now the law in all 50 states (Beresford 1999). However, certain cultural groups continue to resist the concept, most notably the Orthodox Jewish community. They have been particularly effective at lobbying for religious exemptions to the law. In New York physicians are required to make "reasonable accommodation" for patients and families who object to the diagnosis of death on the basis of brain failure. New Jersey goes even further, and provides a legal exemption to Orthodox Jews who refuse to accept brain death (Olick 1991; Olick et al. 2009).

DIAGNOSTIC CRITERIA

The UDDA provides general criteria for determining death, but states that "A determination of death must be made in accordance with accepted medical standards." The first set of standards developed by medical consultants to the

President's Commission were published almost simultaneously with the Commission's report on defining death (Guidelines for the Determination of Death 1981). They described the specific tests that must be performed and fulfilled to meet the criteria. These have been refined several times over the years by a number of medical organizations, leading to a variety of "authoritative" statements that are not entirely consistent with each other. Nevertheless, the essential elements are fairly uniform, and are summarized in Table 3-1.

The diagnostic tests may be summarized in two parts: first, the physician must demonstrate the cessation of all functions of the entire brain; and second, the cessation of these functions must be shown to be irreversible.

At a simplistic level, the central nervous system can be divided into three main components: the cerebrum (or upper brain), the brainstem, and the spinal cord. (The cerebellum is an additional component, but for purposes of this discussion is not distinguished from the cerebrum and brainstem.) The testing performed to examine function of the cerebrum is clinical and fairly crude, consisting primarily of showing that the patient appears to be both unresponsive and unreceptive to noxious (i.e., painful) stimuli, such as applying pressure over the sternum or to the thumbnail. The testing performed on the brainstem is much more technical and specific. Here the physician tests the pupillary reflex (whether the pupils constrict in response to light), the corneal reflex (whether the patient blinks when the cornea is touched with a cotton swab), the oculocephalic reflex (whether the eyes move when the head is turned from side to side), the oculovestibular reflex (whether the eyes move when ice water is injected into the ear canals on both sides), and the oropharyngeal reflex (whether the patient coughs when a suction catheter is passed down the patient's endotracheal tube and stimulates the lining of the airway at the level of the carina).

Table 3-1. DIAGNOSTIC REQUIREMENTS FOR THE DETERMINATION OF BRAIN DEATH

Cessation of Function	Irreversibility
Cerebral: Unresponsivity and unreceptivity	The cause must be known and must be sufficient to explain findings (if not, need confirmatory tests)
Brainstem:	
Pupillary light, corneal, oculocephalic, oculovestibular, oropharyngeal reflexes Apnea test	Rule out drug intoxication Rule out hypothermia Rule out shock Observe 6–24 hours
Spinal cord: loss of function *not* required	

A critical component of the examination, and one that is often performed improperly, is the apnea test. The purpose of this test is to determine if the respiratory centers in the brainstem are responsive to the stimulus provided by a high level of carbon dioxide in the blood. In performing this test, it is important to follow specific protocols to be sure that factors that might depress the brainstem are absent, including hypoxia (a low level of oxygen in the blood), hypotension (a low blood pressure), and hypothermia (a low body temperature). Taking appropriate precautions, the physician removes the patient from the ventilator and allows the level of carbon dioxide in the blood to rise from its normal level of 40 torr to greater than 60 torr. If the patient does not breathe at a carbon dioxide level of greater than 60 torr, then the patient has fulfilled the apnea requirement for the diagnosis of brain death.

The cutoff at 60 torr is recognized as being somewhat arbitrary, which has some interesting implications. There are a number of case reports, particularly in children, in which patients have been legally diagnosed as dead by the standard criteria, only to begin breathing again when their carbon dioxide level inadvertently increased (Vardis and Pollack 1998; Brilli and Bigos 2000). This typically has occurred in the interval between the diagnosis of brain death and the onset of organ procurement, such as when a patient is inadequately ventilated during transport from the intensive care unit (ICU) to the operating room. These cases are important because they show that patients may satisfy the criteria for diagnosing "brain death" but subsequently manifest brain functions incompatible with the diagnosis.

The spinal cord is the third component of the central nervous system. Whereas the Harvard criteria of 1968 assumed that brain death should include the death of the spinal cord, when the criteria were refined in 1981 this requirement was dropped. It might be argued that the spinal cord should never have been considered a part of the brain per se; nevertheless, the potential for continuing function of the spinal cord in the context of a diagnosis of brain death has led to an interesting phenomenon in the literature on brain death known as the Lazarus sign (Dosemeci et al. 2004). This sign typically occurs during the apnea test, when (for reasons that are not entirely clear) neurons in the spinal cord begin to discharge. In its most dramatic form, this spinal cord activity can be quite coordinated, and can result in the patient literally sitting up in bed. Although criteria for brain death specifically state that the Lazarus sign is compatible with the diagnosis of brain death, the possibility of this phenomenon does influence physicians in deciding whether to invite family members to the bedside during the testing for brain death. On the one hand, it can be convincing to show families that the patient is in a deep coma and has no drive to breathe; on the other hand it can be quite awkward if you have to explain how a person who has just sat up in bed is really dead.

In addition to showing that the functions of the cerebrum and brainstem have ceased, it is also necessary to show that this cessation is irreversible. First, and most importantly, this requires having a plausible explanation for the clinical findings [such as a computed tomography (CT) scan of the brain showing massive brain injury]. The brain death literature is replete with papers describing the "false" diagnosis of brain death in patients who had an overdose of a sedative medication that gave them all of the clinical features of brain death, but whose condition was entirely compatible with normal survival after the medication wore off. In truth, these are not "false" diagnoses of brain death (in the sense of showing the inadequacy of the criteria) but rather inaccurate diagnoses of brain death (in the sense that the clinicians failed to fulfill one of the critical requirements of the testing). In addition to having a plausible cause for the findings, physicians must also rule out the presence of other reversible conditions, including testing for known sedative agents and ensuring that the patient is not hypoxic, hypotensive, or hypothermic. Finally, most criteria also require that these findings persist over a period of time (generally 6–24 hours), which requires repeating the entire battery of tests after the specified interval.

A common misperception is that the diagnosis of brain death requires demonstrating that the patient has a "flat electroencephalogram (EEG)," or the absence of brain waves. Although some countries do include this requirement, the diagnosis of brain death is generally considered a "clinical diagnosis" that can be performed entirely by examination at the bedside and without complex technical equipment, except in situations in which the clinical examination may be unreliable (such as in young children or in patients who have received sedative medications). In these cases, a variety of different tests have been proposed to supplement the clinical examination, including the EEG, cerebral blood flow testing, brainstem-evoked potentials, Doppler flow studies, and many others.

Although most of the testing for brain death is fairly innocuous, one aspect is ethically problematic. The apnea test, involving the process of allowing the carbon dioxide level to increase from 40 torr to more than 60 torr, not only provides a powerful stimulus to the respiratory centers in the brainstem, but also may cause significant dilation of the arteries carrying blood to the brain, thereby increasing the pressure in the brain. Because the most common mechanism of brain damage in these patients is the increased pressure caused by brain swelling related to the brain injury, this further increase in pressure has the potential to seriously aggravate and accelerate the brain injury. For this reason, the apnea test should always be the last test performed as part of the brain death examination, and done only if all of the other tests are consistent with brain death. Nevertheless, it is not uncommon for a patient to breathe during the first attempt at apnea testing (showing that the patient is not brain dead), but then to be apneic during a repeat attempt a short time later. The unanswerable question is whether the progression toward brain death was part of the natural progression of the patient's brain injury or whether this further deterioration was actually precipitated by the testing itself.

ARE BRAIN-DEAD PATIENTS REALLY DEAD?

A useful approach to exploring the ethical and philosophical problems with the diagnosis of brain death is through the question, "Are patients who meet brain-death criteria really dead, and if so, then why?" This is the most fundamental question we can ask about the concept of brain death, and indeed it is difficult to imagine how the concept could ever have become widely accepted without a convincing explanation for why satisfying the criteria for "brain death" constitutes death of the human being. To make the point more sharply, imagine the development of criteria for determining kidney death, followed by the claim that these criteria should be sufficient for determining the death of a human being. Clearly such a claim would require establishing a link between the death of a particular organ and the death of the human being. Unfortunately, and perhaps surprisingly, in the case of brain death this link has never been established.

As noted above, the physicians who developed the criteria for brain death (in both the United States and the United Kingdom) offered no argument as to why severe neurological damage causing irreversible coma and inability to breathe spontaneously should be accepted as a criterion of death. By claiming that the diagnosis of brain death signified the complete destruction of the entire brain, they implied that brain death was physiologically equivalent to anatomical decapitation. Brain death was therefore presented in the literature as a "scientific" fact that did not rely upon cultural, religious, or philosophical assumptions. The early research on brain death focused, therefore, upon developing scientific diagnostic criteria for determining when the brain had been completely destroyed.

Brain Death as a Destroyed Brain

Complete destruction of the brain could refer to either structural or functional destruction. Some have insisted that it should refer to structural destruction, since only then could the possibility of brain function (now or in the future) be eliminated (Byrne et al. 1979). Indeed the idea of brain death first arose in the context of the brain liquefaction that often occurs in severely brain-injured patients receiving mechanical ventilation, a phenomenon referred to as "respirator brain" (Dagi 1992).

It is undoubtedly true that the total loss of brain structure necessarily leads to the loss of brain function. When a scientist homogenizes a rat's brain in a blender, no one would believe that continued functioning of that brain is even remotely possible. The loss of function associated with lesser degrees of destruction, however, is often difficult to predict. The brain is a remarkably plastic organ, particularly in childhood. Children with severe epilepsy, for example, may have all of one cerebral hemisphere removed with only subtle loss of brain function. Because the loss of function associated with loss of structure is so unpredictable, some authors have insisted that brain death be defined in terms of "total" brain destruction. Although this standard would surely provide convincing evidence of the loss of brain function, it would be impossible to meet from a practical point of view, since this condition could be confirmed only at autopsy. A condition that could be diagnosed only after death could never be a condition for declaring death.

Nevertheless, if a particular constellation of clinical signs could be identified that invariably correlated with total brain destruction at autopsy, then this set of criteria could be used as a reliable surrogate for determining brain death. However, in a study of 503 cases involving both coma and apnea (including 146 autopsies studied for neuropathological correlation), "it was not possible to verify that a diagnosis made prior to cardiac arrest by any set or subset of criteria would invariably correlate with a diffusely destroyed brain" (Molinari et al. 1980).

More recently, this finding was confirmed in an autopsy series of 41 patients who fulfilled clinical criteria for brain death. Only "mild" changes of neuronal ischemia and necrosis in one-third of the cerebral hemispheres and about one-half of the brainstems were reported. In other words, in this modern study of the brains of patients diagnosed as brain dead, in many parts of the brain the majority of the neurons still appeared to have been alive at the time of death. They concluded that "Neuropathologic examination is therefore not diagnostic of brain death" (Wijdicks and Pfeifer 2008).

If brain death constitutes death, but does not correlate with a structurally destroyed brain, then perhaps it correlates with the complete loss of all brain function. This is, in fact, the requirement specified in the UDDA, which stipulates that brain death is the irreversible absence of all functions of the entire brain, including the brainstem.

The UDDA does not define the process for testing these functions, but instead leaves this question to be determined by "accepted medical standards." Yet the standards that have been developed hardly test for all of the functions of the brain; indeed, they are highly selective and incomplete, targeting primarily those brain functions that are easy to assess by a bedside clinical examination. For example, the brain functions associated with consciousness are assessed simply by seeing if the person is responsive to commands or painful stimulation. Today we know that some patients diagnosed as in a vegetative state who appear to be unconscious on clinical examination show evidence on functional magnetic resonance imaging (fMRI) scanning of being capable of complex cognitive functioning (Monti et al. 2010). Given the severity of brain injury seen in most patients diagnosed as brain dead, we think the potential for any conscious awareness in these patients is remote; our point is only that the clinical methods used in brain death examinations to assess for consciousness are now known to be inadequate in many cases.

Aside from consciousness, brain death testing involves examination of a variety of brainstem reflexes, as discussed above, while ignoring a number of critical brain functions, such as the regulated secretion of pituitary hormones. Neurologist James Bernat (1992, 2006a) has defended the current standards on the grounds that they test for all of the "critical" functions of the brain, yet this does not seem to be the case. Although the brainstem reflexes that are tested are easy to elicit during a bedside examination, none of them (except for the apnea test) involves any function critical to survival. Conversely, the current standards do not test for brain functions that are critical for survival, such as the regulated secretion of hormones that control the body's fluid and salt balance, or the brain mechanisms that control body temperature. Indeed, multiple studies show that many (and in some studies most) patients diagnosed as brain dead actually retain brain function related to these hormones (Fackler and Truog 1987; Truog and Fackler 1992; Halevy and Brody 1993; Shewmon 1997; Truog 1997). In light of these studies, it is clear that a clinical diagnosis of brain death does not coincide with cessation of all the functions of the entire brain and therefore does not, strictly speaking, constitute "physiological decapitation." Although Shewmon has pointed out that some patients do manage to survive even without these hormonal brain functions, this merely calls into question whether *any* of the brain's functions are actually critical for survival, as will be discussed below (Shewmon 2001).

Furthermore, the issue of temperature control presents a Catch-22 conundrum. The standards for diagnosing brain death require that the patient be warm at the time of testing in order for the results to be valid, yet maintenance of normal body temperature is itself a brain function. Hence one of the requirements for making the diagnosis of brain death—that the patient be warm—strictly speaking actually rules out the diagnosis.

More controversial have been studies showing that many brain-dead patients continue to show EEG activity on testing of their brain waves. Whether this represents true function or merely random uncoordinated electrical activity is unknown, but in at least some cases the activity appears compatible with at least semiconscious functioning (Rodin et al. 1985). Also controversial is how to interpret data showing that brain-dead patients have a significant rise in both heart rate and blood pressure at the time the incision is made to procure transplantable organs. Although this may suggest that brain centers involved in the perception and response to pain are still functioning, it may be that these responses could be mediated entirely at the level of the spinal cord, which would make them compatible with the diagnosis of brain death (Shewmon 2001).

In sum, whereas the UDDA states that brain-dead patients must have the irreversible absence of all functions of the entire brain, the standards include testing for only very selective functions that can be evaluated at the bedside, most of which are not physiologically critical for survival. Furthermore, the testing ignores functions that are physiologically critical, and when these functions have been evaluated, they are often found to be present. Quite literally, the criteria for diagnosing brain death do not meet the legal standard in a large number of cases. Even the most ardent supporters of the brain-death criterion acknowledge these findings (Bernat 1992, 2006a).

These problems highlight the fact that all efforts to make brain death a scientifically valid concept have been doomed to fail in the absence of any unifying theory as to why brain death is death. No "gold standard" for making the diagnosis has ever been established. Shewmon notes that by 1978, over 30 different diagnostic criteria for brain death had been published, none of them validated, and without any consensus on the concept itself or the diagnostic "gold standard" (Shewmon 2009). Literally hundreds of articles have been published in the medical literature evaluating different methods for making the diagnosis of brain death, including cerebral angiography, radionuclide scanning, Doppler ultrasonography, brainstem-evoked potentials, and so on. But the absence of a gold standard for the diagnosis of brain death makes this entire literature uninterpretable.

For example, one study examined the use of P-31 MR spectroscopy in 24 patients declared brain dead on the basis of standard clinical criteria plus EEG testing. All but one showed no cerebral energy metabolism. Yet when this patient "survived" for more than several weeks, the authors concluded that she could not "really" have been brain dead in the first place (even though she fulfilled all the diagnostic criteria), and thereby declared their new diagnostic method a perfect success (Kato et al. 1991). By making the "gold standard" a moving target, dubious new technologies are compared against dubious old technologies, and the literature on the subject ends up being both incoherent and unintelligible.

Brain Death as the Prognosis of Cardiac Arrest

In 1981 Bernat and colleagues published a seminal paper entitled "On the definition and criterion of death," in which they developed the idea that brain death is equivalent to death because it represents "the permanent cessation of functioning of the organism as a whole" (Bernat et al. 1981). The origins of this idea came from the early literature on brain death, which relied heavily on the view that brain death was an acceptable definition of death because brain-dead patients were doomed to suffer a cardiac arrest (and a traditional death) within a short period of time, regardless of the intensity of life support provided.

In recognizing the problems involved in trying to define brain death in terms of the anatomical destruction of the entire brain, Korein wrote that "it is not required that every neuron in the brain be destroyed. Rather, it implies that the extent of destruction and consequent irreversible neuronal dysfunction is so great that regardless of any supportive measures, irreversible cardiac arrest and death of the adult human brain is inevitable within one week" (Korein 1978, cited in Gervais 1986, 7). Similarly, the cooperative study of cerebral death conducted by investigators from the National Institutes of Health between 1972 and 1975 sought to define brain death as that constellation of neurological findings that results in cardiac arrest within 3 months (Collaborative Study 1977). This line of reasoning was also cited as a justification for not requiring the use of tests that cannot be performed in a bedside examination (such as electroencephalography or studies of cerebral blood flow), since "If [clinical tests] are 100% specific for non-viability, why wait for another study?" (Morray et al. 1987).

This line of reasoning—that brain death is death because it accurately predicts the development of a cardiac arrest—is rather obviously flawed from a logical perspective. It conflates a prognosis with a diagnosis, and thus confuses the process of dying with the state of death. We can imagine many severe and advanced clinical conditions in which the prognosis for a cardiac arrest within a short period of time is almost certain. Patients with such conditions can clearly be said to be dying, but it makes no sense to claim that they are already dead. It can be difficult to understand how otherwise sophisticated clinicians and scientists could have made such a fundamental mistake. Moreover, available evidence (reviewed in the next section) does not support the thesis that a diagnosis of brain death is inevitably followed within a short period of time by cardiac arrest.

Brain Death as the Loss of Integration

Bernat and colleagues used the data on the prognostic significance of brain death to advance the first comprehensive theory of why brain death is a justified criterion of death. They proposed that death should be defined as "the permanent cessation of functioning of the organism as a whole" (Bernat et al. 1981).

Bernat asserts that this functioning manifests itself as the emergent properties of the organism: "The organism as a whole comprises that set of functions that are greater than the mere sum of the organism's parts" (Bernat 2006a). This theoretical construct sought to correct what they viewed as a major flaw in the language of the UDDA, which seemed to imply that there are two distinct definitions of death, one based on circulatory–respiratory functions and the other based on neurological functions. They offered a unified definition of death that could be fulfilled by different sets of criteria, including those based on the loss of either circulatory–respiratory or neurological functions.

We believe that Bernat and colleagues are correct in seeking a unified definition of death, and we agree that death should be defined biologically in terms of the cessation of functioning of the organism as a whole. (As will become clear in Chapter 5, we hold that the cessation of functioning defining death should not only be permanent but irreversible.) We disagree, however, that the neurological criteria for determining death fulfill this standard.

Today very few patients who are diagnosed as brain dead have prolonged somatic survival, for the simple reason that once their families are informed of the diagnosis they are either removed from the ventilator immediately or after they donate vital organs for transplantation. In this regard, somatic death after the diagnosis of brain death has become a self-fulfilling prophesy. But the work of Shewmon and others has clearly demonstrated that brain death need not be prognostic of somatic death, and that the brain is not necessary for the continued functioning of the organism as a whole. Shewmon (1998) reported on 175 cases in the literature of patients with a formal declaration of brain death who survived for more than 1 week. He found that their survival probability decreased exponentially in two phases, the first with a half-life of 2–3 months, followed at 1 year by a slow decline to more than 14 years (Shewmon 1998).

This is consistent with many case reports in the literature of brain-dead patients who have been kept alive on mechanical ventilation for prolonged periods of time. Most commonly this has occurred with women who were pregnant at the time they were diagnosed as brain dead, when their families wanted them to be maintained on life support until their fetuses could reach a gestational age compatible with delivery (Powner and Bernstein 2003; Lane et al. 2004). In other cases, family members have elected to keep their brain-dead loved ones at home on mechanical ventilation, fed through a gastrostomy tube. In the most dramatic case, initially described as part of Shewmon's series, a boy who became brain dead at the age of 4 years from meningitis survived for more than 20 years at home. At the time of his death, autopsy showed an entirely calcified brain, with no neural elements visible either grossly or microscopically (Repertinger et al. 2006).

Given all of the early data indicating that brain death was highly prognostic of somatic death, how do we explain the more recent findings of Shewmon and others? Shewmon has provided a logical explanation for the historical misunderstanding about the prognostic significance of brain death. Physiologically, brain death is analogous to high cervical cord transection, since both result in the nearly complete disruption of the brain's control or influence over the body (Shewmon 1999, 2001, 2004). In cervical cord transection, the loss of modulatory input from the brain to the body is initially very disruptive, often resulting in a life-threatening form of hemodynamic instability known as "spinal shock." In the absence of the medications and monitoring capabilities of the modern ICU, patients with spinal shock rarely survive, explaining the findings observed with brain-dead patients in the 1960s and 1970s.

With the development of the modern ICU, however, it became possible to better support patients through the acute period following either brain death or high cervical cord transection. Indeed, a significant part of the survival benefit of modern ICU care comes from the use of technologies that function as a "surrogate brainstem," regulating those brainstem functions related to hemodynamic and respiratory homeostasis that are critical to life. Once this acute phase has passed (generally a month or two after the injury), the body develops the capacity to self-regulate, and if provided with minimal "surrogate brainstem" functions (such as mechanical ventilation and supplemental hormones), can survive for many years.

Pushing the point even harder, Shewmon has described how most of the brain's functions are not directed toward integration of the organism, and how most of the integrative functions of the body do not require brain function. The following is a list of integrated functions, from Shewmon (2001), that are *not* mediated by the brain and are possessed by at least some patients diagnosed as brain dead:

- Homeostasis of a variety of mutually interacting chemicals, macromolecules, and physiological parameters, through the functions especially of the liver, kidneys, and cardiovascular and endocrine systems, but also of other organs and tissues (e.g., intestines, bone and skin in calcium metabolism, and cardiac atrial natriuretic factor affecting the renal secretion of rennin).
- Elimination, detoxification, and recycling of cellular wastes throughout the body.
- Energy balance, involving interactions among liver, endocrine systems, muscle, and fat.
- Wound healing, the capacity for which is diffuse throughout the body and that involves organism-level, teleological interaction among

blood cells, capillary endothelium, soft tissues, bone marrow, vasoactive peptides, and clotting and clot lysing factors (maintained by the liver, vascular endothelium, and circulating leukocytes in a delicate balance of synthesis and degradation).
- Fighting of infections and foreign bodies through interactions among the immune system, lymphatics, bone marrow, and microvasculature.
- Development of a febrile response to infection.
- Successful gestation of a fetus in a brain-dead woman.
- Sexual maturation of a brain-dead child.
- Proportional growth of a brain-dead child.

Can we therefore conclude that it is possible for organisms to continue to function "as a whole" in the absence of brain function? We believe yes, but first must address an important objection to this conclusion. This is the claim that patients who meet the neurological criteria have lost the capacity to breathe, and that without continued respiration they do, in fact, manifest the loss of functioning of the organism as a whole.

This mistakenly presumes that the conceptually important aspect of integration of the organism as a whole is the natural source of the functions rather than the functions themselves (Wikler 1984, 170). For example, individuals with the permanent cessation of renal function have lost integrative functioning, and will soon die unless that function is replaced by artificial dialysis. Similarly, an individual who suffers the acute onset of complete heart block (from myocarditis, for example) has also lost integrative functioning and will soon die unless treated with an artificial pacemaker. Even a patient with severe hypothyroidism has lost integrative functioning and will soon die unless treated with artificial thyroid hormone. Nor is there anything special about breathing. Patients with high level cervical quadriplegia are unable to breathe without mechanical ventilation. Assuredly, all of these individuals are alive, and they retain integrative functioning because the necessary functions persist with artificial support. In other words, the fact that integrative functions are supplied or supported artificially is irrelevant to the determination of whether individuals are alive. Similarly, we argue that brain-dead patients remain alive and continue to breathe, in the sense that air continues to move into and out of their lungs, despite the fact that this function is being supplied artificially.

Somewhat paradoxically, Bernat himself has endorsed this view, writing "[W]ithin an organism, there is an important distinction between a function and the mechanism that performs that function. . . [W]hat is important for a death criterion is whether a function is being performed adequately, not necessarily how it is being performed. In the context of death determination using a circulation formulation, for example, what is important is the absence of respiration and circulation, not the absence of heartbeat and spontaneous breathing" (Bernat 1998). Bernat uses this argument as evidence of the importance of the brain, since it cannot be replaced by a machine. This is true, but it doesn't follow that brain-dead bodies are dead on the basis of a biological definition of death. This quote also endorses our view that integration of the organism can continue, even if a ventilator is necessary to maintain the function of respiration.

The evidence seems irrefutable that humans can retain the integrated function of the organism as a whole even in the absence of brain function. Moreover, whether integrative functioning lasts for only a few minutes or hours after a diagnosis of brain death, the body is not dead (according to a biological definition) as long as the integrative functioning continues. Yet Bernat and others have continued to hold the view that patients who are brain dead fail to show integrative functioning, despite evidence of prolonged survival. Was the boy in the case report described above—who over 20 years grew from a child into an adult, digested food, and excreted waste—actually dead for those two decades?

Bernat would say yes, and insist that this child was dead since the age of 4 years, based on his view of what counts as "critical functions of the organism as a whole." In a defense of brain death, he wrote that "Examples of critical functions of the organism as a whole include (1) consciousness, which is necessary for the organism to respond to requirements for hydration and nutrition; (2) control of circulation, respiration, and temperature control, which are necessary for all cellular metabolism; and (3) integrating and control systems involving chemoreceptors, baroreceptors, and neuroendocrine feedback loops to maintain homeostasis. Death is the irreversible and permanent loss of the critical functions of the organism as a whole" (Bernat 1998). Because the brain-dead patients with prolonged survival described by Shewmon and others fulfill the second and third criteria, the implication of his claim is that an organism cannot have integrated functioning if it does not have the capacity for consciousness.

Bernat has steadfastly been defending both the concept of brain death and the definition of death as the cessation of functioning of the organism as a whole for almost 30 years, but unfortunately at this point his arguments reach a cul-de-sac from which there is no escape. On the one hand, if he holds that the capacity for consciousness is necessary for the continued functioning of the organism as a whole, then he is logically committed to the view that at least some patients who have been diagnosed as being in a vegetative state, and who have permanently lost consciousness, are dead. This is a view he has consistently denied. Moreover, on the basis of a biological conception of life and death, it is far from clear why the capacity for consciousness is a necessary condition for life, as this is not present in plants, lower forms of animal life, and the early stage human fetus. On the other hand, if he were to concede that integrated functioning is possible in the absence of consciousness, then he must acknowledge that at least some brain-dead patients are still alive. It is logically inconsistent for both claims to be true.

Bernat and others want to have it both ways, because for some purposes they want to define death in terms of integrated functioning, but at the same time they want to accord a special status to the brain. The notion that the brain is the "critical system," the organ that is indispensible to maintaining the body's integrated functioning, has long been a popular view, and was the position taken by the President's Commission in their 1981 report. But the data that have accumulated over the past several decades clearly show that this view is false.

The distinctions between the neurological- and circulatory–respiratory-centered criteria for determinations of death are summarized in Table 3-2 (Truog and Robinson 2003; Truog 2007). The purpose of the comparison is to make the point that the only salient feature that differentiates living persons from brain-dead patients is the capacity for consciousness. If patients currently diagnosed as brain dead are dead, then it is because they have lost the capacity for consciousness, not because they have lost the functioning of the organism as a whole.

The view that the diagnosis of death should be based on whether patients are capable of manifesting aspects of consciousness is known as the "higher-brain" criterion. This view appeals to our sense that the brain is the most important organ for making us who we are as persons. The brain is the one organ that cannot be replaced by artificial technology, and is essential for enabling the experiences that make life worth living. In the Chapter 4 we discuss in

Table 3-2. COMPARISON OF FEATURES OF LIVING PERSONS WITH THOSE DIAGNOSED AS DEAD BY NEUROLOGICAL VERSUS CIRCULATORY–RESPIRATORY CRITERIA

Features of Living Persons	Living Persons	Dead by Neurological Criteria	Dead by Circulatory–Respiratory Criteria
Heart-beating, warm, well-perfused	Yes	Yes	No
Breathing	Yes	Yes (with ventilator)	No
Functioning vital organs (liver, kidneys, etc.)	Yes	Yes	No
Capable of reproducing	Yes	Yes	No
Capacity for consciousness	Yes	No	No

detail the "higher-brain" standard of death that focuses upon the capacity for consciousness.

Certainly human beings have many characteristics that give them a unique niche within the living world. But with regard to maintaining integrated functioning, humans are much like other forms of life in the animal and plant kingdoms, most of which maintain integrated functioning without a conscious brain or a "critical system." Instead of relying upon a premiere organ, the integrative functions of these plants and animals are distributed diffusely, rather than being localized. Shewmon has helpfully drawn an analogy to holograms, in which destruction of a part of the image does not result in the loss of localized information (as would be the case with a photograph). Instead, this damage results in a slight degradation of the image overall. Similarly, focal structural losses in an organism generally result in diffuse changes, with functioning that is less efficient and coordinated than before (Shewmon 2001). Life is truly an emergent phenomenon, more than the sum of its parts, but one that is not dependent upon the functioning of any single organ or system, not even the brain.

THE CIRCULATORY–RESPIRATORY CRITERIA AND INTEGRATED FUNCTIONING

As indicated above, we endorse the biological definition of death as the irreversible cessation of the functioning of the organism as a whole. From a biological perspective, living organisms are distinct from the inanimate world by virtue of their use of energy-consuming processes to maintain homeostasis, defined as "the ability of an organism to maintain a constant internal environment by regulating its physiological processes and by making adjustments to the external environment" (Macklem and Seely 2010). A recent exploration of this concept suggested that life may better be defined in terms of the concept of homeokinesis: "the ability of an organism to utilize external energy sources to maintain a highly organized interval environment fluctuating within acceptable limits in a far from equilibrium state" (Que et al. 2001; Macklem and Seely 2010). The laws of thermodynamics indicate that entropy is always increasing; the universe is continually moving in the direction of greater randomness and disorder. Living organisms are discrete pockets of activity within this universe in which this process is reversed—or at least kept in check—with energy drawn from the environment. Once these energy-consuming processes stop, the organism begins to disintegrate, ultimately rejoining the "dust" of the inanimate world. We assert that organisms continue to function as a whole as long as these homeostatic, homeokinetic entropy-resisting processes continue, and that death occurs at the moment when the entropy-increasing forces have irreversibly exceeded those that are resisting this process. Although it may be difficult, or even impossible, to determine empirically exactly when this moment occurs, theoretically it does occur at an instant in time. As such, we assert that death is an event, not a process.

The notion that the definition of death could be tied to thermodynamic concepts was explored by Julius Korein as early as 1978 (Korein 1978). His theory asserted that the brain was the "critical system" of the body, because it was the only system that could not be replaced by artificial means, and because "when brain death . . . occurs, irreversible cardiac arrest will inevitably follow regardless of the maintenance of all resuscitative procedures," always within a week and usually within 24–48 hours (27). Although we accept his general theory about the relevance of thermodynamic concepts to defining death, we now know that his beliefs about the prognostic significance of brain death are not true, and that there is no one "critical system" in the body.

Two energy-consuming functions that are essential to maintaining homeostasis and the functioning of the organism as a whole are circulation and respiration. Circulation can be understood as the process that brings nutrients to the cells of the organism and carries away wastes. Respiration is the process of gas exchange that occurs across the cellular membranes, involving the uptake of oxygen and the release of carbon dioxide in animals, and the reverse in plants. These two processes function across a broad swath of the living world, from single-cell amoebae to humans. Single-cell organisms need no systems to assist with respiration and circulation, since they are able to effect these exchanges with the environment directly. But as organisms become more complex, they need transport mechanisms for gases and nutrients. In humans, of course, these functions are provided by the respiratory and the circulatory systems.

As discussed above, determinations of life and death depend upon the whether the functions are being performed, not the mechanism by which they are performed. For example, in patients with heart or lung failure, the functions of circulation and respiration can be accomplished by a heart-lung machine (known as ECMO, or extracorporeal membrane oxygenation). Patients on ECMO can be fully alive, in the sense of continuing to possess both circulation and respiration, even though their hearts and/or lungs may be completely destroyed. ECMO can theoretically support life for an indefinite period, although practically its use is usually limited to several weeks because of associated complications such as bleeding and infection.

In sum, we propose that death be defined as the moment at which the integrated functions of the organism as a whole irreversibly cease, as determined by when the forces tending to increase entropy irreversibly overcome those that are opposing it. Furthermore, the emergent properties that give rise to this integrated functioning depend upon sustained circulation and respiration, and irreversible cessation of these functions is therefore a sufficient criterion for declaring death. As described in more detail below, an advantage of this formulation is that it can be applied across a broad range of the biological world, including organisms that do not have consciousness, or even brains.

NEUROLOGICAL VERSUS CIRCULATORY–RESPIRATORY CRITERIA FOR DETERMINING DEATH

Supporters of a neurologically centered standard for determining death assert that this has always been the implicitly accepted standard, and that the traditional emphasis upon circulatory and respiratory functions has merely been an indirect method of testing for the absence of brain function. The claim has been that brain death is not an essentially new way of determining death, but merely a more refined and sophisticated way of diagnosing when death has occurred. As Howard Brody has explained, "The reason heart and lung function became the legal and social standard to determine the time of death, we might argue, is that when one either stopped breathing or suffered cardiac arrest, irreversible loss of total brain function invariably followed within minutes. Today, however, mechanical devices have made it possible to maintain artificially heart and lung function even in the presence of brain death. If we have other tools, such as the Harvard criteria, to tell us what is actually going on with the brain, we should rely on those, and not the artificially maintained heart and lungs, to determine death" (Brody 1981, 79). For professionals who may be uncomfortable with a relatively new definition of death, there may be a sense of security in believing that we are simply applying traditional criteria in a more sophisticated context. In addition, there is an intuitive appeal to the idea that the declaration of death has always been a statement about the status of the brain, and that we have focused upon the loss of circulatory and respiratory activity only because they have invariably been (up until recently) reliable indicators of the loss of brain function.

But the view that our definition of death has always been brain centered may be a distorted interpretation of the historical facts. As Veatch has countered, "It would take fancy philosophical footwork to claim that the shift from a heart-oriented definition to a whole-brain-oriented definition involved no fundamental conceptual shift, but those who take this position have given no argument to support it nor provided any explanation for the empirical evidence that many individuals consciously maintain that individuals with dead brains and beating hearts are alive" (Veatch 1992). The recent furor over the fate of Terry Schiavo revealed that a large segment of the American population believes that patients like her are not only alive, but possess a life worth living, suggesting that they regard circulation and respiration as having significance beyond the support they provide to consciousness and brain function. Indeed, the growth of organ donation using donation after circulatory determination of death (DCDD) protocols (described in detail in Chapter 5) also undermines the claim that death has always been (or is even currently) seen as a purely neurological phenomenon, since in this context death is determined solely on the basis of circulatory criteria, without any assessment for whether the donors are neurologically dead.

BRAIN DEATH AND THE PRESIDENT'S COUNCIL ON BIOETHICS

A recent attempt to explain "brain death" within the context of a biological definition of death is presented in a remarkable document, a white paper of the President's Council on Bioethics entitled "Controversies in the Determination of Death," published in 2008 (The President's Council 2008). The work, the first of its kind since that of the President's Commission in 1981, has been called courageous, in the sense that it took an honest, probing, and critical look at 40 years of scholarship and legislation around the concept of brain death (Shewmon 2009). This report rejected all of the previously advanced rationales for a neurological standard of death. In particular, it rejected the reigning view that brain death is death because it represents the loss of the integrated functions of the organism as a whole. After reviewing all of the integrated functions retained by brain-dead patients, it concluded that "If being alive as a biological organism requires being a whole that is more than the mere sum of its parts, then it would be difficult to deny that the body of a patient with total brain failure [the Council's term for 'brain death'] can still be alive, at least in some cases" (57).

The Council fully understood the profound influence that this conclusion could have on the life-saving practices of organ donation and transplantation. And so, perhaps to avoid these consequences, it proposed yet another rationale for why brain-dead patients should be considered dead.

The Council adopted "total brain failure" to describe this condition, which is an improvement over "brain death," as it does not beg the question of whether patients with this clinical presentation are in fact dead. However, it is also a misnomer; as we have seen, patients with this clinical diagnosis typically do not manifest the failure of all brain functions. Although the Council made a valiant and novel attempt to preserve neurological criteria for determining death in the context of a biological conception of death, we argue that their position is incoherent.

A telltale sign of incoherence in the defense of the neurological standard is the bizarre language that is invoked to support it. For example, The Council states that "The machine [mechanical ventilator] is, in essence, ventilating a corpse—albeit one that in many ways does not look like a corpse" (3). Similarly, the "brain-dead" patient is a "heart-beating cadaver" (8). Reviewing the clinical presentation of "total brain failure," the Council notes that patients with this condition display aspects of "somatic health" (39). The language gets particularly strained at this point: "If the body is a cadaver, then, of course, it is no longer fitting to speak about its 'health.' Nonetheless, *something like health* is still present in the body of a patient with this diagnosis" (39). How can even something like health be present in a cadaver? Finally, the report describes "cases of prolonged 'somatic survival' after 'whole brain death'" (45). The persistent use of scare quotes signifies that something fishy is going on.

Perhaps, however, the linguistic oddity merely reflects the distinction between appearance and reality in this perplexing domain. Patients determined to be dead by neurological criteria certainly don't appear to be dead, as they are breathing and warm to the touch. But appearances can be deceptive, and our language may reflect appearances that conflict with reality—for example, we continue to speak of the sun setting. Early in the Council's report, it echoes the President's Commission by noting that "The apparent signs of life that remain—a beating heart, warm skin, and minimal, if any, signs of bodily decay—are a sort of mask that hides from plain sight the fact that the biological organism has ceased to function as such" (3). Yet it is the latter fact that is disputed by critics of determining death according to established neurological criteria; for, as illustrated above, the biological organism represented by the "brain-dead" patient continues to function in a variety of significant ways. In view of this continued biological functioning of the organism as a whole, on what basis can we distinguish the appearance and the reality of being alive? Why are the beating heart, warm skin, and lack of bodily decay merely the appearance of life? Moreover, how can a corpse gestate a fetus? More than 20 years ago, Englehardt (1986) offered a succinct challenge to, if not definitive refutation of, this alleged distinction between appearance and reality. Regarding brain-dead bodies, he observed that "They appear to be alive because they are in fact alive. It is because human biological life continues unabated that transplant surgeons are interested in such bodies as an ideal source for harvesting organs" (209). In sum, if the cessation of vital functioning of the organism constitutes death, it is difficult to escape the conclusion that patients diagnosed with "total brain failure" are not dead.

Nevertheless, the President's Council endorses a biological conception of death (49–52) and wrestles with the at least apparent incoherence between the bodily functions maintained by patients with "total brain failure" and the determination that they are dead. It includes a table, entitled "Physiological Evidence of 'Somatic Integration'" (56), listing the variety of biological functions maintained by patients with "total brain failure" with the aid of mechanical ventilation and other measures of support. The Council explicitly parts company with the President's Commission on the rationale for determining death by neurological criteria. This philosophical departure is announced in the following passage: "But, as we have seen, even in a patient with total brain failure, some of the body's parts continue to work together in an integrated way for some time—for example, to fight infections, heal wounds, and maintain temperature. If these kinds of integration were sufficient to identify the presence of a living 'organism as a whole,' total brain failure would not serve as a criterion for organismic death, and the neurological standard enshrined in the law would not be philosophically well-grounded" (60).

The Council attempts to escape this impasse in explaining why patients with total brain failure are dead by making a very significant step, that is, by abandoning integration of the organism as the key concept in defining death and also abandoning "the false assumption that the brain is the 'integrator' of vital functions" (60). Instead, the Council appeals to the novel notion of "the vital *work* of a living organism—the work of self-preservation, achieved through the organism's need-driven commerce with the surrounding world" (60). The living organism does its vital work when it satisfies the following three criteria: it exhibits (1) "receptivity to stimuli and signals from the surrounding environment," (2) "the ability to act upon the world to obtain selectively what it needs," and (3) "the basic felt need that drives the organism to act as it must, to obtain what it needs" (61).

The white paper claims that patients with a diagnosis of total brain failure completely fail to meet each of these criteria. In contrast, it asserts that patients in a persistent vegetative state (PVS), who breathe spontaneously but show no signs of consciousness, completely fulfill these criteria. Let us suppose that these criteria of vital work discriminate between the living and the dead. For this account to be persuasive, the contrast between these two groups of patients must be transparent. The explication of these three criteria of vital work is skimpy, making it difficult to determine whether they apply to patients with "total brain failure." We find it far from clear that these patients entirely lack the ability to respond to their environment, in view of the range of vital functions that they can perform, such as fighting infections and wound healing. In addition, the vital functioning of these patients may also be understood as satisfying the second criterion of acting upon the world to obtain selectively what they need. More generally and importantly, the range of biological functions displayed by patients with total brain failure would seem to testify to their continued ability to do the vital work of self-preservation, albeit with the aid of mechanical ventilation.

Although the capacity for spontaneous breathing of patients with PVS is emphasized as indicative of their being alive, it is also noted that mentally intact patients with cervical spinal cord injuries may lack this capacity, and thus require mechanical ventilation; however, they assuredly are alive. This entails that the lack of spontaneous breathing on the part of patients with total brain failure cannot count as making them dead. Nor is it clear why the permanent loss of consciousness makes them (biologically) dead, given the range of organismic functioning that they maintain.

Summing up its philosophical position, the Council asserts, "If there are no signs of consciousness and if spontaneous breathing is absent and if the best clinical judgment is that these neurophysiological facts cannot be reversed, Position Two [endorsed by the Council] would lead us to conclude that a once-living patient has now died" (64). We submit that this conclusion is a *non sequitur*. According to the Council, neither loss of the capacity for consciousness (as in PVS) nor loss of the capacity for spontaneous breathing (as in cervical quadriplegia) by itself makes a patient dead. Why, then, does the combination of losing both these capacities constitute death in patients with total brain failure when a host of other biological functions of the organism as a whole are maintained? In short, once again, a coherent account of why individuals diagnosed as having "total brain failure" are dead has not been supplied.

To their credit, however, the Council was blunt about the consequences if their account were ultimately deemed unconvincing: "*If* indeed it is the case that there is no solid scientific or philosophical rationale for the current 'whole brain standard,' then the only ethical course is to stop procuring organs from heart beating individuals" (12, emphasis in original). Although we agree with the premise that there is no solid scientific or philosophical rationale for treating "total brain failure" as constituting death, we disagree with the Council's conclusion that failure to find an adequate justification for neurological criteria for determining death means that organ donation from heart-beating individuals must stop. Instead, in Chapter 6, we provide an alternative foundation on which to build an ethical framework for continuing the life-saving practices of organ donation and transplantation, one that does not depend upon neurological criteria for determining death or the "dead donor rule."

BRAIN DEATH AND CLINICAL PRACTICE

At the beginning of this chapter we noted that physicians are trained to believe that the diagnosis of brain death is scientifically based on empirical and objective criteria, just like the diagnosis of a myocardial infarction. On the one hand, much of medical practice is in accord with this dogma, such as when physicians cite the time of death on death certificates as the time when brain death testing was complete, rather than the time when circulatory–respiratory function ceased.

On the other hand, both research and anecdotal accounts suggest that physicians and other clinicians continue to harbor doubts about whether brain death is really death. Perhaps one of the most telling signs is the continued use of the label itself. Despite efforts by transplantation advocacy groups to encourage physicians to speak simply of "death" rather than "brain death," the persistent use of the term suggests that clinicians view it as distinct from a traditional understanding of death.

A study by Youngner and colleagues from 1989 showed considerable ambivalence about the meaning of the diagnosis of brain death (Youngner et al. 1989). In this study of physicians and nurses who were involved in organ procurement and transplantation, only 35% were able to correctly identify the legal and medical criteria for determining death. More specifically, most did not believe that brain-dead patients are "really" dead, but felt comfortable with the process of organ procurement because the patients are permanently unconscious and/or imminently dying. Although some have taken this study to be evidence that we simply need to do a better job at educating clinicians about the "facts" of brain death, the editorial that accompanied this paper observed that this confusion was "appropriate," given the ambiguities inherent in the concept itself (Wikler and Weisbard 1989).

Another interesting insight comes from a debate in the European literature among anesthesiologists about whether brain-dead patients should receive an anesthetic during organ procurement procedures. Some argued that because many, if not most, brain-dead patients retain some brain functions, we cannot be sure that they are incapable of experiencing some pain during the surgery, even if only at a rudimentary level (recall the data showing that brain-dead donors do show a significant rise in heart rate and blood pressure at the time that the surgical incision is made). According to this logic, they argued that the patients should be given an anesthetic, even if only to be "on the safe side." Others disagreed. Surprisingly, their position was not based on the claim that the patients were incapable of experiencing pain. Instead, they were concerned that if the public learned that anesthesiologists were giving an anesthetic to "dead" patients, it would make them suspicious that the patients were not really dead. Essentially they were arguing that the risk of undermining the trust and confidence of the public in the organ transplantation enterprise was a greater concern than the risk of not giving an anesthetic to a patient who might retain the capacity to feel some pain (Dalgleish 2000; Keep 2000; Matta 2000; Poulton and Garfield 2000; Young and Matta 2000).

But perhaps one of the most revealing insights comes from an anecdote. In June 2005 Larry King was covering a tragic story for CNN about a 26-year-old woman who suffered a massive hemorrhage into an undiagnosed brain tumor while she was pregnant, leading to the diagnosis of brain death (King 2005). She was maintained in an ICU on life support for almost 3 months until she delivered a little girl at 27 weeks gestation. On the show Larry King interviewed Dr. Sanjay Gupta, a practicing neurosurgeon and medical reporter for CNN. The transcript from the show reads as follows:

> **Larry King**: And, Dr. Gupta, we should explain again, in your— medically, is a brain-dead person dead?
>
> **Dr. Sanjay Gupta**: Well, you know, a dead person really means that the heart is no longer beating. I mean, that's going to be the strict definition of it. So a brain-dead person is someone who has no chance of recovery, has no brain function, is requiring artificial support to be alive, but people do draw a distinction between brain dead and dead. This is where the whole field of organ transplantation sort of came to be, Larry, based on that distinction.
>
> **Larry King**: So in other words, you wouldn't transplant an organ from Susan?
>
> **Dr. Sanjay Gupta**: Well, you actually could, because she is brain dead. Her brain is not going to recover. If that was a choice that was being made, you could actually transplant an organ from a brain-dead person into someone else.

As a neurosurgeon, Dr. Gupta is certainty very familiar with the criteria for diagnosing brain death and with the implications of that diagnosis, and yet when perhaps caught a little bit off-guard, he expressed views very similar to those of the clinicians in Youngner's study, views that are completely "wrong" with regard to the dogma surrounding the meaning of brain death.

In this interchange, Dr. Gupta erroneously claimed that the "strict definition" of death is when "the heart is no longer beating," and that brain death refers primarily to a prognosis ("no chance of recovery"), rather than a diagnosis. Whereas he emphasized that the distinction between brain dead and dead was how "the whole field of organ transplantation came to be," the field has actually been built on the claim that these two are equivalent. Not surprisingly given this description, Larry King assumed that Susan Torres could not be an organ donor, at which point Dr. Gupta correctly stated that she could be. He implied that this would be permissible because "her brain is not going to recover," not because she was actually dead.

This view is not unusual. Tracy Schmidt, then the Executive Director of Intermountain Donor Services, has noted that "many individuals would donate the organs of a loved one who was severely brain-damaged . . . even if their loved one does not fulfill all of the specific criteria for 'brain death,'" and that "[a]t times, physicians are willing to declare 'brain death' when a patient has not fully met the criteria for brain death outlined by the American Academy of Neurology, but the physicians know from their clinical experience that the individual has no chance of survival" (Schmidt 2004).

In sum, although there are many who claim that the concept of brain death is now accepted worldwide, we need only to scratch a little below the surface to uncover a great deal of ambivalence about how this criterion relates to the diagnosis of death. Perhaps no one has captured this ambivalence more concisely than a judge in Florida, who in a comment about a brain-dead patient stated: "This lady is dead and has been dead and she is being kept alive artificially" (*New York Times*, December 5, 1976, cited in Green and Wikler 1980).

CONCLUDING REMARKS ON BRAIN DEATH

The upshot of our lengthy investigation of established brain-based criteria for determining death is that the functioning of the brain, by itself, has nothing to do with whether human beings are alive or dead, any more than any other individual organ. The brain is not the integrator of the human organism, without which it ceases to maintain homeostasis and lapses into entropic disintegration. Nor is the brain necessary to perform "the vital work" of the organism. Hence, human beings rendered brainless by massive neurological injury, or even by decapitation, are not dead as long as their bodies continue to function as an organism with the aid of technological intervention. In this regard, brain failure is no different from kidney failure. Just as dialysis permits life to continue despite dysfunctional kidneys, so do intensive care interventions permit a "brain dead" body to remain alive (and even to gestate a fetus). Although the brain is necessary for consciousness, consciousness is not necessary to life, and the permanent absence or loss of consciousness does not constitute human death. The human being dies when the body ceases to function as an organism, which is marked by the irreversible cessation of circulation and respiration.

We contend that these conclusions are inescapable as long as we posit a biological conception of death. In other words, it is a matter of *fact* that "brain-dead" individuals are not dead, though this fact is relative to a biological conception of death. Bernstein, in a recent account of philosophical pragmatism, makes this point about the relativity of facts in a general way: "There *are* facts of the matter, even though these facts are relative to the adoption of a conceptual scheme—and even though alternative conceptual schemes may be incompatible with each other" (Bernstein 2010, 161). These conclusions about the brain and death certainly will be rejected by those who understand human life and death as based on the concept of what it means to be a person or what counts as being distinctively human in a metaphysical sense that transcends or departs from biology. In Chapter 4 we investigate critically the "higher-brain" standard of death, which is the leading alternative conceptual scheme in terms of which human death is defined.

4

Challenges to a Circulatory–Respiratory Criterion for Death

In Chapter 3 we argued that the concept of brain death is inconsistent with a biological conception of death based on the functioning of the organism as a whole, and that therefore we should rely solely on the traditional criteria for determining death on the basis of circulatory and respiratory functioning. In this chapter we continue to explore the connection between death and the brain by considering brain-based objections to the traditional criteria for determining death and then discussing critically an alternative brain-based standard of death based on the concept of personhood and the capacity for consciousness.

BRAIN-BASED OBJECTIONS TO CIRCULATORY–RESPIRATORY CRITERIA FOR DETERMINING DEATH

Advocates of determining death on the basis of neurological criteria have argued that the traditional standard for determining death faces insuperable objections and must be rejected because it leads to absurd conclusions. We consider in this section two objections relating to decapitation and "the division scenario."

The Decapitation Gambit

Circulatory and respiratory criteria for determining death imply that a decapitated human being or other type of animal would be alive so long as it maintains circulatory and respiratory functioning (Lizza 2009a, 2009b). Lizza declares that this is absurd: "if anything entails one's death, decapitation certainly does, despite whatever artificial support might be given to sustain one's decapitated body as an integrated organism. Thus, if we are willing to accept decapitation as death, we should also be willing to accept physiological decapitation (total brain failure) as death" (Lizza 2009a).

When unpacked logically, this "decapitation gambit" consists of two closely related arguments, which can be stated formally as follows.

ARGUMENT ONE
1. Decapitation is an infallible sign and sufficient condition of death.
2. It is possible for a decapitated animal to maintain circulatory and respiratory functioning, either spontaneously for a short period of time or with mechanical assistance.
3. The circulatory–respiratory standard identifies the irreversible absence of circulation and respiration as determining death.
4. It follows that the circulatory and respiratory standard must be false as a necessary and sufficient condition for determining death, because premises 1 and 2 entail that an animal dead by virtue of decapitation can maintain circulation and respiration.

ARGUMENT TWO
1. "Brain death" constitutes physiological decapitation.
2. Decapitation is an infallible sign and sufficient condition of death.
3. Hence, individuals diagnosed as "brain dead" are necessarily dead.

Common and central to both of these arguments is the first premise in argument one and the second premise in argument two. Is decapitation an infallible sign of death? As the quote from Lizza suggests, it may seem perfectly obvious that decapitation constitutes death and thus without need for any explanatory rationale. However, several rationales might be provided to support this proposition. First, it is self-evident. Second, everyone agrees that a decapitated animal is dead. Third, it has been universally adopted by authoritative commentators within Orthodox Judaism as an infallible sign of death. Fourth, in view of the role of the brain in integrating the functioning of the organism as a whole, a decapitated animal without a brain is necessarily dead. Finally, the permanent absence of consciousness signifies death of the human being, and a decapitated human body lacks the organ responsible for consciousness.

We contend that the first four rationales are either logically or empirically deficient and thus fail to establish that a decapitated animal is necessarily dead. The fifth rationale does not count as a refutation for the position that advocates sole reliance on circulatory and respiratory criteria for determining death. The crucial problem with the decapitation gambit is that it is doubly question-begging. It begs the question in arguments one and two by assuming that decapitation is necessarily death. It also begs the question in argument two by assuming that "brain death" is physiological decapitation. Our discussion above regarding brain functions retained by individuals diagnosed as "brain dead" indicates that this condition is not equivalent to physiological decapitation. Nevertheless, we will set this aside to focus on whether decapitation necessarily coincides with death.

Is it self-evident that decapitation signifies death? One reason why it may seem self-evident, or at least obvious, is that decapitation is a method of causing death in the context of human execution and animal slaughter, after which the victim rapidly progresses to an inanimate corpse. But is the decapitated animal invariably dead *at the moment* when decapitation occurs? It is necessary to answer this question in order to avoid conflating a diagnosis with a prognosis of death, which we criticized in Chapter 3. To be on a trajectory of no return with death as the inevitable and imminent outcome is not the same as being dead. Assuming a biological definition of death, if integrated functioning of the organism as a whole can be maintained following decapitation, even for only a few moments, the organism may be imminently dying but is not yet dead. Decapitation normally sets in motion a process of disintegration of the organism as a whole. Absent technological efforts to maintain circulation and respiration, all biological functions integrated or mediated by the brain will necessarily cease. It doesn't follow that the organism as a whole has become entirely *disintegrated* at the moment of decapitation. We will take up below the issue of whether observed activity of the decapitated animal represents mere reflex or other biological activity of isolated parts of the organism and not the integrated functioning of the organism as a whole.

Think of the proverbial farmyard scene of a chicken with its head cut off running around before collapsing. Is this a dead chicken on the move? This case challenges the claim of self-evidence as well as the proposition that everyone agrees that a decapitated animal is dead. It seems counterintuitive to declare that the moving chicken is already dead, rather than dying and soon to be dead. Likewise, it seems natural to describe the chicken as dropping dead when it collapses. It is important, however, to recognize that such intuitions may be mistaken. What appear to be signs of continued life in the decapitated animal might reflect only biological activity of particular disconnected organs, not the integrative functioning of the organism as a whole. Although possible, this conclusion does not seem compelling to us. Although it moves aimlessly, the chicken's ability to run and to flap its wings suggests integrated activity of the headless body. Although the brain has been severed from the body, the spinal cord remains intact and provides the neural input necessary to drive the integrated behavior of running. Whether this degree of integration is sufficient to conclude that the chicken continues to manifest the "integrated function of the organism as a whole" may be debatable; however, the question of whether the chicken is alive or dead turns upon a judgment about the degree of this integration, not upon the mere fact that the chicken is decapitated.

Within Orthodox Judaism, decapitation has been regarded as a certain sign of death (Rosner 1999). Some scholars within this tradition have invoked the analogy between decapitation and brain death, with the latter seen as physiological decapitation. Because the decapitated animal is dead, brain death constitutes death of the human being. Yet other Orthodox scholars have contested the brain death diagnosis as a sign of death because respiration continues with the aid of mechanical ventilation (Kunin 2004). In the context of this debate, two Israeli investigators conducted an experiment involving a decapitated pregnant sheep intended to validate decisively a neurological standard for determining death (Steinberg and Hersch 1995). This experiment helps to shed light on the force of the decapitation gambit.

Perhaps the most striking challenge to accepting "brain death" as death of the organism as a whole is the known capability of pregnant women diagnosed with this condition to gestate a viable fetus for a considerable period of time, followed by successful birth of a living infant. How can a dead body possible accomplish this feat? The Israeli experiment was designed to prove that this is possible.

A pregnant near-term sheep was anesthetized and connected by intubation to a respirator. Dissection of the head exposed the carotid arteries, which were tied and cannulated. The sheep's head was fully cut off and the endotracheal tube placed in the tracheal opening. Pharmacological measures were introduced to maintain blood pressure and heart rate. Thirty minutes after decapitation, a healthy lamb was delivered by caesarian section (Steinberg and Hersch 1995).

The investigators drew the following conclusion from their experiment. "Our experiment has proved that a decapitated animal in an intensive care set-up is capable of maintaining normal circulation and a normally beating heart. Moreover, we have proven that a decapitated animal can serve as an incubator for her fetus, and that a normal newborn can be delivered despite the demise of its mother, if appropriate modern measures are taken. There is no doubt that a completely decapitated animal is a dead animal; nonetheless, all vital organs, including a fetus, can function normally in such a situation."

Logically, the investigators were able to reach this conclusion only by virtue of assuming the premise that "There is no doubt that a completely decapitated animal is a dead animal." They stated furthermore that "A decapitated animal is by all logical, theological, and philosophical criteria a situation of clear organismal death." Yet they supplied nothing beyond these question-begging assertions to back up the proposition that a decapitated animal is necessarily dead.

We contend that this experiment proves the very opposite of what was intended. The fact that the investigators were able to maintain circulation and respiration in a decapitated sheep, along with continued gestation of the fetal lamb for 30 minutes, indicates that vital functioning of the organism as a whole can be preserved despite decapitation, with the aid of mechanical ventilation and pharmacological intervention. For those who believe that pregnant "brain dead" women who can gestate a fetus in the intensive care setting must be alive, this experiment provides no evidence to the contrary. Instead, it demonstrates that decapitation is not incompatible with life.

As discussed above, a decapitated animal that maintains temporary heart beating or is able to briefly run around presents an ambiguous situation; based on a biological conception of death, some might consider the animal alive and others as dead. This is not the case for the sheep experiment, in which the decapitated animal clearly showed continued signs of homeostatic functioning reflecting integration of the organism as a whole. Based on a biological conception of death, there is no ambiguity here: the sheep remained alive during the experiment.

Finally, appeal to decapitation as death on account of permanent loss of consciousness cannot refute sole reliance on circulatory and respiratory criteria for determining death. The latter position adopts a biological definition of death; the former defines death with respect to a conception of personhood or what is considered essential philosophically to *human* life (as distinct from merely biological existence). There are reasons for and against these conceptually distinctive definitions of death, but the decapitation gambit and the analogy between brain death and decapitation are not decisive considerations in favor of a consciousness-based standard, which we discuss below.

As we have argued, decapitation does not necessarily signify death, understood as the cessation of functioning of the organism as a whole. Only if it did, would the decapitation gambit refute a biological conception of death that appeals solely to circulatory and respiratory criteria for determining death. The decapitation gambit fails. Setting aside any preconceptions about whether decapitation constitutes death, the sheep experiment proves that a decapitated animal can continue to live with the aid of technological intervention.

Division Scenario

A related objection to a biological conception that adopts circulatory and respiratory criteria for determining death invokes the "division scenario" (Khushf 2010). Imagine the following ghoulish thought experiment. A homeless man named John, sleeping in a park, is approached by an evil scientist who injects him with an anesthetic agent. John is taken to the scientist's laboratory where his head is severed and attached to life support equipment able to maintain circulation and respiration and brain functioning within the severed head. Simultaneously, the headless body is attached to separate life support equipment, which maintains biological functioning. In an article defending the "whole brain" criterion for determining death, Khushf (2010) describes an abstract version of this division scenario (without the narrative details), which he sees as refuting the "nonbrain position on death."

According to Khushf, a biological conception of death that relies on circulatory and respiratory criteria implies "the absurdity (from the perspective of a policy on human death) that two individual organisms might arise by dividing one" (Khushf 2010, 24). Additionally, he argues that this conception of death is not able to endorse the intuitively obvious judgment that the individuality of the person whose head has been severed but remains conscious and responsive is preserved in the severed head and not in the headless, but still breathing, body. Playing the scenario out further, Khushf writes, "let the head say 'please don't turn me off,' and despite protestations, we turn it off. We now ask: is the 'individual' or 'organism' still alive? I think nearly everyone would say 'no, the individual died when the animated head was no longer perfused'" (24). He concludes that "[t]he division scenario can thus be taken as a conclusive refutation of a nonbrain account" (24).

Does Khushf's critique hold up? It clearly would be absurd to describe the division scenario in a way that makes the individual John identical with both the severed head and the headless body. For this contradicts the meaning of "an individual being," which can't be identical with two distinct beings. The nonbrain account of death that we endorse does not imply this absurdity. We agree that the person John now inhabits the severed head in the thought experiment above; whereas John's headless, and personless, body remains alive as a separate being. We see no absurdity in this. When John's life support is stopped, John dies—the person or individual named John ceases to exist. But John's separated body continues to live, albeit in a brainless, vegetative state. Of course, normally a living person and a living person's body are continuous, which makes this account of the division scenario bizarre, but not absurd. In contrast, there is nothing bizarre in distinguishing a person's living body from the person who has ceased to exist.

It might also seem absurd to understand the division scenario as one person splitting into two persons. (We describe this as apparently absurd because we are not convinced that it is absurd but will assume that it is for the sake of the argument.) If a nonbrain account of death were to equate a living human being with a person, then it would imply this apparently absurd conclusion. Our biological conception of death does not assume a one-to-one correspondence between living human beings and persons. Indeed, it is meant solely to determine when a human being has died and makes no claims about either personal identity or personhood.

Is there one human being or two human beings in the division scenario? We see two living beings—a conscious severed head and an unconscious headless body, which are both alive because they are hooked up to life support equipment that maintains circulation and respiration. It might seem a stretch to describe either of these dismembered beings as a *human* being, though less a stretch for the head than the headless body. Yet each, on our account, is a living being, and it doesn't seem absurd to describe each as biologically a human being. A living human being can cease to be a person, as is undoubtedly true of the headless but still breathing body. We also regard the "brain dead" body as no longer a person despite being alive. (This latter judgment is not dictated by a biological conception of death. We will see below in a discussion of the "higher brain" standard of death that some who adopt a biological conception of death understand the "brain dead" individual as not only alive but still a person.) Thus the division scenario constitutes a situation in which a living human being who is a person becomes split into two living beings: John, the individual person, remains alive in the severed head, and John's body remains alive without being inhabited by a person.

As indicated above, Khushf thinks it absurd "that two individual organisms might arise by dividing one." Before challenging this, we need to address the issue of whether the division scenario can be reasonably understood as resulting in two organisms. It is difficult to be confident in characterizing such bizarre scenarios. We might take the position that neither the severed head nor the headless body is an organism, though we find it not unreasonable to regard both as organisms. The headless body maintained on life support is not a single organ but a system of organs that maintains integrative homeostatic functioning. Likewise, the severed head is not merely a single organ, but consists of a brain, eyes, nose, ears, and mouth, all of which, in accordance with the thought experiment, continue to function such that this living being produces sensory experience and communicative speech. Thus, we see no absurdity in interpreting the division scenario as resulting in two human organisms. What is bizarre is not necessarily absurd. In other contexts, the division of one organism into two is neither bizarre nor absurd. A single human embryo can divide into two monozygotic twins. In sum, as long as the distinction is made between a living human being and a person, the biological conception of death that adopts circulatory and respiratory criteria for determining death has no difficulty in making sense of the division scenario.

HIGHER BRAIN STANDARD OF DEATH

We have rejected the determination of death on the basis of a diagnosis of "brain death" because some brain functioning continues in individuals diagnosed with this condition and, more importantly, because these individuals manifest functioning of the organism as a whole, making this diagnosis incompatible with a biological definition of death. The concept of whole brain death has also been criticized from an entirely different perspective, which appeals to personhood and the loss of consciousness as the key to human death. In the early 1970s some scholars, espousing what has come to be known as "the higher brain standard of death," criticized the emerging conception of whole brain death on two grounds: (1) its advocates had failed to explain coherently why individuals with irreversible coma and inability to breathe spontaneously were dead; and (2) death of the entire brain is not necessary to determine the death of the human being (Veatch 1975; Englehardt 1975). Proponents of the higher brain standard argue that individuals diagnosed as "brain dead" are dead because they have permanently and irreversibly lost the capacity for consciousness, which puts an end to their lives as *human* beings. Since consciousness has been thought to be lodged in the higher portion of the brain—the cerebral cortex—death of the entire brain, including the brainstem, is not necessary for human death.

For many, especially philosophers, this "higher brain" standard for determining death is appealing. Although it has not been endorsed as a legal standard for determining death in any jurisdiction, and was rejected by two U.S. public bioethics commissions that addressed the issue of determining death, it deserves careful consideration, especially in view of the failure to explain the rationale for the whole brain standard of death in terms of a biological definition of death. Because individuals diagnosed as "brain dead" retain an impressive array of functioning of the organism as a whole, either they are not dead, as we contend, or they are dead for reasons other than the cessation of biological life. If they are not dead, then either we need to put a stop to our current practices of procuring vital organs from these individuals while their hearts continue to beat, or we need a different ethical approach to vital organ donation that does not depend on the dead donor rule (DDR). One of the potential virtues of the higher brain standard is that, if defensible, it can provide a rationale for continuing to procure organs from "brain-dead" but heart-beating donors that preserves the DDR. These donors are dead not because their bodies have ceased to function but because they have irreversibly lost the capacity for consciousness, which is alleged to be essential for being alive as a human being.

In this section, we provide a critique of the higher brain standard, which discusses both conceptual difficulties and practical problems with its application. Our aim is not to undertake a comprehensive philosophical examination of the higher brain standard, as this would require a foray deep into metaphysical territory, which is beyond the scope of this book.

Conceptual Issues

Just as "whole brain death" is a misnomer in view of the preservation of some brain functioning in many patients diagnosed as "brain dead," so the "higher brain" standard is semantically misleading in suggesting that the key function of consciousness is lodged in the neocortex. Neurologists Machado and Korein (2009, 200) have recently observed that "consciousness does not bear a simple one-one relationship with higher or lower brain structures and, consequently, the higher brain view is wrong, because the definition 'consciousness' does not harmonize with the anatomical substratum 'neocortex.'" In a detailed examination of animal and human studies, Merker (2007) argues that the upper brainstem can generate consciousness without a functioning cerebral cortex. Perhaps most interesting in this regard are case reports of the behavior of children with hydranencephaly (Shewmon et al. 1999; Merker 2007). These children are born with fluid in place of the cerebral cortex. Yet when raised in a nurturing environment, they are able to move around and navigate in a manner indicative of visual perception, respond to sounds and faces, and thus to interact with others, though lacking the ability to speak. In short, they are conscious despite having no cerebral cortex. Shewmon, who carefully examined and observed two such cases, notes that "The hydranencephalic children proved that the cortical doctrine of consciousness was simply not true in a congenital situation" (Shewmon 1997, 58). Damasio (2010, 82), drawing on Shewmon's observations, echoes this view: "The condition [hydranencephaly] gives the lie to the claim that sentience, feelings, and emotions arise only out of the cerebral cortex."

These observations about the anatomical location of consciousness might suggest no more than a semantic infelicity in "the higher brain standard" locution, which therefore ought to be replaced by some other term, such as the "consciousness-based standard." (For the sake of convenience we will continue to use the "higher brain standard" terminology, as it is entrenched in the literature.) Yet this semantic issue points to a serious practical problem that we discuss in detail below. Advocates of the "higher brain" standard have presumed the anatomical location of consciousness in the cerebral cortex (e.g., McMahan 2002, 423–455; Glannon 2007, 148–177) and, more significantly, have been rather cavalier about diagnosing the absence of consciousness, which is critical to the application of this definition of death. The fact that a functioning cerebral cortex is not necessary for consciousness has important implications for thinking about patients in a persistent vegetative state (PVS) who have sustained massive injury to the higher brain and are judged to lack consciousness on the basis of clinical examination. These individuals have been considered dead on the higher brain standard despite an intact brainstem that permits them to breathe spontaneously.

McMahan, one of the most philosophically sophisticated advocates of a con-sciousness-based standard of death, observes, "[i]t is an accepted tenet of neurol-ogy that a patient in a PVS occasioned by the destruction of the cerebral cortex altogether lacks the capacity for consciousness or mental activity. If this is true—and one can be reasonably confident, though not certain, that it is—then brain death cannot be the criterion for the loss of the capacity for consciousness" (McMahan 2002, 427). Although acknowledging a lack of certainty, McMahan proceeds to describe with confidence individuals with PVS as dead by virtue of irreversible loss of consciousness. But do we know that they lack consciousness? The term "higher brain standard" erroneously fosters the idea that consciousness is necessarily lodged in a certain part of the brain, such that destruction of, or widespread injury to, that part irreversibly causes the loss of consciousness. This formulation of a standard of death in terms of damage to a particular brain loca-tion arguably has diverted attention from the critical issue of assessing the absence of consciousness, without which the "higher brain standard" has no more than theoretical interest. We discuss the status of PVS patients in detail below.

Consciousness is identified as the key to life and death by advocates of the higher brain standard because they see it is as essential to what it means to be a person. Although what it takes to be a person is far from clear, the ability to experience self and others—subjectivity and intersubjectivity—is generally thought to be an essential attributes. Accordingly, any consciousness-based standard for determining death necessarily parts company with a biological conception of death. Plants and lower animals are not persons, nor is the human fetus before the development of the neural capacity for consciousness. But these beings certainly are alive. Why should death be something essentially different on the human level than in the rest of the biological realm? Feldman has posed this challenge with respect to the following three sentences:

1. JFK died in November 1963.
2. The last dodo died in April 1681.
3. My oldest Baldwin apple tree died during the winter of 1986.

Feldman remarks, "If 'died' were used in different senses in these sentences, then the inference would be an eyebrow-raiser. It would be a play on words; it would be like the case in which a man tells us he owns two planes: one a single-engine Cessna that he uses on business trips and the other a single-bladed Stanley that he uses in his woodworking shop" (Feldman 1992, 19).

Advocates of the higher brain standard have replied to this challenge by noting that death is not a univocal concept. We naturally speak of the death of persons, just as we speak of the death of organisms; however, the former is not identical to the latter. McMahan argues that we have two concepts of death, and that this is consistent with commonsense. In support of this he notes that "[w]hen the body of Nancy Cruzan died in 1990, after spending almost eight years in a persistent vegetative state (PVS), her family, who had gone to the Supreme Court in their efforts to terminate the body's life support, engraved on her tombstone: 'DEPARTED JAN 11, 1983/AT PEACE DEC 26, 1990'" (McMahan 2002, 423). In other words, the death of the person who was Nancy Cruzan occurred several years prior to the death of her body. We are not convinced that the meaning of this inscription supports McMahan's view—if *she* was dead on January 11, 1983, why did she have to wait until December 26, 1990 to be at peace? In any case, there is no incoherence in recognizing two concepts of death. Yet there is a linguistic oddity in this position that may sow confusion. We naturally speak of death without qualification—not dead as a person versus dead as a body, but just dead. Without being careful, it is easy to conflate the issue of whether someone has a humanly significant life with the question of whether the individual is alive. We suggest below that this conflation may underlie the lack of concern with diagnosing consciousness that characterizes advocates of the higher brain standard.

A more serious, and arguably fatal, conceptual problem is that there is no consensus on what counts as being a person (Wikler 1984). Some see human fetuses as persons; others do not. Jonas, an early critic of "brain death," described the new conception of death as "a curious revenant of the old soul-body dualism. Its new apparition is the new dualism of brain and body. In a certain analogy to the former it holds that the true human person rests in (or is represented by) the brain, of which the rest of the body is a mere subservient tool. . . . My identity is the identity of the whole organism, even if the higher functions of personhood are seated in the brain. How else could a man love a woman and not merely her brains?" (Jonas 1974, 139). In other words, for Jonas, the death of the brain does not constitute the death of the person, despite the loss of the "higher functions of personhood." Echoing Jonas, Shewmon remarks that "to equate human life and death with the presence or absence of consciousness is to recapitulate the Cartesian error. . . If a brain lesion were to impede the exercise of mental faculties, even permanently, the person becomes seriously disabled but does not therefore cease to be a living human being or to be substantially the same person" (Shewmon 1997, 72).

We do not take sides on this debate about whether the "brain dead" remain persons, though we are inclined to agree that they have lost personhood. But the positions of Jonas and Shewmon are neither incoherent nor otherwise irrational.

In any case, it seems at least desirable, if not necessary, that the underlying rationale for the concept of death and the criteria of its application, by virtue of which we sort the living from the dead, be amenable to universal agreement. Everyone agrees that a stone cold corpse is dead. Not everyone agrees that a warm, breathing, but permanently unconscious body is dead or has ceased to exist as a person. In contrast, the biological definition of death has universal applicability—everyone agrees that a body has died when the functions of the organism as a whole have ceased, as marked by the body's irreversible absence of respiration and circulation. (There may be disagreement about the exact specification of criteria for determining death based on this biological definition.) Not so for a consciousness-based conception purporting to define when a person has died. In a wide ranging critique of the concept of personhood as it relates to the issue of moral status, Beauchamp diagnoses the problem at issue here: "[l]iterature on the criteria of persons is mired in intractable dispute in a wide range of cases, including fetuses, newborns, the irreversibly comatose, God, extraterrestrials, and the great apes. Facts about these beings are not the source of the dispute. The problem is created by the vagueness and the inherently contestable nature of the ordinary language concept of person" (Beauchamp 1999, 319).

Practical Difficulties

We view the conceptual problems highlighted above, especially the lack of agreement on what counts as the loss or absence of personhood, as raising serious, if not insurmountable, challenges to the higher brain standard of death. The burden of proof is greatly increased by practical difficulties in applying this conception of death.

PVS

As we have indicated, advocates of the higher brain standard of death have regarded individuals with a diagnosis of PVS as dead by virtue of permanent and irreversible loss of consciousness. PVS is caused by profound neurological damage, either from traumatic injury or loss of oxygen to the brain. These patients are characterized as "awake but not aware." Though showing no reliable signs of consciousness, PVS patients display sleep–wake cycles, with their eyes open while awake. The diagnosis is made on the basis of clinical examination with respect to three criteria: "(1) no evidence of awareness of the self or the environment; (2) no evidence of sustained, reproducible, purposeful, or voluntary response to auditory, tactile, or noxious stimuli; and (3) no evidence of language comprehension or expression" (Monti et al. 2009, 82). It is noteworthy that this diagnosis is highly unreliable. In a review article, Bernat describes an "alarmingly high rate of error in diagnosis of vegetative state reported in two series of patients admitted to rehabilitation units, in which 37% and 43% of patients purportedly in vegetative state were identified on careful testing to have measurable awareness" (Bernat 2006c, 1183). These data should give pause to proponents of the higher brain standard; for, obviously, measurable awareness denotes at least primitive consciousness.

Although patients correctly diagnosed as in PVS show no signs of conscious response to stimuli on clinical examination, scientific knowledge is lacking to prove that the brain damage they have sustained makes them incapable of conscious experience. For example, the assumption that vegetative patients are unable to experience pain is open to question. As Shewmon observes, "PVS patients often grimace to noxious stimuli and manifest primitive withdrawal responses. Advocates of the cortical theory write off such behaviors as mere brainstem or spinal reflexes, but that dismissive attitude is based more on an a priori assumption than a scientific conclusion" (Shewmon 1997, 60). How could we ever be confident that pain-like behavior in these patients is not accompanied by any aversive feeling?

More generally, Panksepp and colleagues argue that in addressing the question of consciousness in PVS patients it is important to distinguish conscious affective states from cognitive awareness of such feelings (Panksepp et al. 2007). They note that "[t]here really is no well-conceived reason as to why subcortical brain structures should not be able to generate unreflective affective states and basic experiences of homeostatic drives such as thirst or hunger. . . . The fact that in PVS patients damage to cortex and thalamus is more pronounced than damage to lower brain areas strongly suggests that such raw affective states could still be experienced by patients in a vegetative state" (Panksepp et al. 2007, 6–7). And if these patients can experience pain or discomfort, then obviously they can't be dead on the basis of lacking capacity for consciousness.

Moreover, Shewmon argues that it is impossible to be certain that PVS patients lack consciousness. Describing the medical consensus that PVS patients lack awareness, he observes, "[n]eurologists (and everyone else) had fallen obliviously into the logical fallacy that mere *absence of evidence* constitutes *evidence of absence*. No one seemed to be concerned that perhaps what is eliminated by cortical destruction might be the capacity for external manifestation of consciousness rather than consciousness itself in other words, that what is called 'PVS' might in reality be merely a 'super-locked-in' state" (Shewmon 1997, 60). Recently, brain imaging studies have strongly suggested a capacity for consciousness in some patients diagnosed as being in a vegetative state

(Monti et al. 2010). Some PVS patients who were asked to imagine playing tennis or moving around a room in their house displayed patterns of brain activation identical to healthy volunteers requested to perform the same mental tasks (Owen et al. 2006; Monti et al. 2010). Yet these patients at the time lacked any detectable awareness on clinical examination. The interpretation that these experiments proved that some patients diagnosed as vegetative display consciousness has been challenged, however (Nachev and Hacker 2010).

On the other hand, these and other experiments suggest that it might be *possible* to develop reliable diagnostic tests for the presence and absence of consciousness using brain imaging; yet this potential is far from being realized. In a recent philosophical account of consciousness, drawing on the latest findings of neuroscience, Noe observes that "at present we are not even close to being able to use brain imaging to get a look inside the head to find out whether there is consciousness or not" (Noe 2009, 18).

One of the reasons why commentators, including advocates of the higher brain standard, so readily describe PVS patients as lacking consciousness may be that this is built into the definition of this condition. However, the absence of detectable signs of consciousness doesn't entail the absence of consciousness. Furthermore, even if brain imaging is performed to confirm the diagnosis, it does no more than investigate correlations between hypothesized patterns of brain activation and stimuli applied to the individual whose brain is being scanned. These stimuli include various mental tasks involving verbal instructions and various interventions to probe sensory awareness. But there is no comprehensive and validated battery of testing, with reliably interpretable results, that taps all possible signs of consciousness, including cognitive and affective awareness. Moreover, functional brain imaging fosters the illusion that scientists can *see* what is going on, or not going on, in the brain; rather, these brain images constitute technically sophisticated constructions from experimental data that permit hypotheses about brain functioning (Dumit 2004; Noe 2009, 19–24). In sum, the gap between absence of evidence and evidence of absence is especially wide and deep in this domain, making diagnosis of death on the basis of lack of consciousness highly precarious.

Some argue that these diagnostic difficulties merely raise practical problems in the application of a consciousness-based standard of death. For example, Lizza acknowledges that it might be necessary, at least for now, to limit determination of death on the basis of irreversible lack of consciousness to a diagnosis of brain death (Lizza 2006, 164–175). However, the logical challenge posed by Shewmon, based on the distinction between absence of evidence and evidence of absence, also applies, at least in theory, to the diagnosis of "brain death." We noted above that the clinical testing for absence of consciousness in making this diagnosis is superficial. Do we *know* beyond the possibility of reasonable doubt that the underlying brain damage that is correlated with this diagnosis makes *any* consciousness impossible? The answer is "Yes" when structural imaging of the brain indicates that it has been liquefied; but not all cases that satisfy the clinical criteria for brain death afford this highest level of certainty. The problem is only compounded by the fact that there is no scientific or philosophical consensus on exactly what consciousness is. In other words, the boundaries of the concept of consciousness are unclear such that there is no agreement on what types of responses to stimuli are indicative of consciousness (Velmans 2009, 330–337). We are not suggesting lack of reasonable confidence that individuals diagnosed as "brain dead" have irreversibly lost consciousness. However, we find it surprising that philosophers who have advocated a consciousness-based standard for determining death seem so little concerned about how to diagnose the absence of consciousness—the very functioning on the basis of which life or death turns according to this position. A definition of death is useless if it is not practically operational with a very high degree of certainty in demonstrating that the criteria for determining death—in this case, the absence of consciousness—have been satisfied.

This cavalier attitude toward diagnosing consciousness suggests to us that the conflation between being alive and having a life that is worth living may be responsible for the lack of concern about the practical applicability of a consciousness-based definition of death. Many are convinced that those who are diagnosed as "brain dead" and in PVS have lost any personally significant life. If so, does it matter if there is some sort of intermittent residual and primitive level of consciousness that is retained? It may not matter if what is at stake is the decision to cease life support, consistent with the prior preferences and values of the incompetent patient. It does matter to the cogency of a declaration of death based on the irreversible loss of consciousness. Some advocates of the higher brain standard might reply that personhood can be lost despite the presence of some low level conscious awareness. Perhaps what is required for personhood, the loss of which constitutes death, is self-consciousness (Rich 1997, 215). However, without diagnostic sensitivity and specificity for self-consciousness, the determination of death on this basis will be impractical.

Even if we could be certain based on expert diagnostic examination that PVS patients irreversibly lacked consciousness (or self-consciousness), determining them to be dead would still be highly counterintuitive for most people. Brain dead individuals are corpse-like in that they are immobile and not responsive, but the fact that they are breathing, have a beating heart, and are warm to the touch makes it difficult to view them as dead. It is all the more difficult to view PVS patients, who breathe spontaneously, as dead. The idea of being dead is paradigmatically associated with being a corpse. The higher brain standard endorses a concept of death of the person that has nothing to do with being a dead body, thus making it incredible for most people. The counterintuitive idea that the PVS patient is dead gives rise to the retort that no one would countenance burying or cremating a spontaneously breathing human body.

Summing Up: Why the Higher Brain Standard Should Be Rejected

Since the early 1980s, scholars have often deployed a three-part analysis of the definition of death in terms of (1) the concept of death, (2) the criteria for determining death, and (3) the tests indicating that the criteria have been satisfied (Bernat et al. 1981). The higher brain standard of death fails with respect to each of these components. This approach defines death in terms of the concept of personhood: a human being is dead when it ceases to exist as a person. As we have noted, the concept of personhood is inherently vague and contested, and there is no agreement on what it takes to be a person or when personhood is lost. The higher brain standard takes the irreversible loss of consciousness as the criterion for determining death. However, the boundaries of the concept of consciousness are unclear. Nor is it clear whether any signs of consciousness in a human being are sufficient to indicate that the person remains alive or whether what counts is absence of higher forms of consciousness, such as cognition and self-awareness. Finally, we have no reliable tests for the absence of consciousness.

In sum, the higher brain standard is neither conceptually clear nor practically applicable. Moreover, it is highly counterintuitive insofar as it classifies as dead spontaneously breathing individuals diagnosed as permanently vegetative, on the assumption that they have irreversibly lost the capacity for consciousness.

DEATH AND ORGAN TRANSPLANTATION

We began our discussion of the higher brain standard in the previous section with the observation that this position appears attractive as a way to preserve the practice of procuring vital organs from heart-beating "brain dead" donors without violating the dead donor rule. They are dead, it is alleged, not because they have ceased to function as organisms but because, lacking the capacity for consciousness, they are no longer alive as persons—the only way of being alive that (allegedly) matters from a human perspective. It is noteworthy that the felt need for a determination of death prior to procuring vital organs is probably the only reason for invoking a higher brain standard of death. As noted in Chapter 1, a diagnosis of death is by no means necessary before legitimately deciding to stop life-sustaining treatment. It is highly unlikely that the appeal to the absence of consciousness, even if reliably diagnosed, would by itself serve to mark the presence of death for any purpose other than organ donation: for example, grieving the loss of life, burial or cremation, accessing life insurance, probating a will, or terminating a marriage. Currently we use traditional circulatory and respiratory criteria for determining death to serve these purposes. To be sure, death certificates for those diagnosed as "brain dead" are dated at the time of the diagnosis, not when life-sustaining treatment is withdrawn. Family members may not recognize their loved ones as dead, however, until the heart beat has ceased. In sum, the higher brain standard is not an all-purpose criterion for determining death.

Moreover, it is not even fully suitable for determining death in the context of vital organ donation. As discussed in Chapter 5, vital organs increasingly are being procured on the basis of circulatory and respiratory criteria after life support has been withdrawn. Although the donor has lost consciousness at the time that death has been declared, it doesn't follow that the absence of consciousness is irreversible. The higher brain standard offers no help in settling the controversial question of whether these donors are really dead, or known to be dead, at a few minutes after their hearts have stopped beating. Accordingly, the higher brain standard, at best, is only of limited utility in underwriting current practices of vital organ donation. Moreover, the conceptual and practical problems with this position seriously challenge any apparent value it may have in upholding organ transplantation under the DDR.

The definition of death has been a topic of bioethical inquiry and debate for over 40 years owing primarily to its presumed central role in justifying organ donation. The problems we have noted in the whole brain and higher brain standards of death suggest that this presumption—that we need to update or change the traditional standard of death in terms of circulatory and respiratory criteria—is misguided. Instead of trying to determine when human beings are dead so that their vital organs can now be donated we need to inquire and debate when it is ethical to procure vital organs from still-living individuals. This is the topic that we take up in Chapter 6, after discussing current practices of vital organ donation after circulatory determination of death in Chapter 5.

5

Donation after Circulatory Determination of Death

Two pathways for vital organ donation currently exist. The first is donation after brain death, in which the donor is declared dead by neurological criteria (as detailed in Chapter 3), permitting the removal of all vital organs, including the heart, under optimal conditions while they are still being perfused with oxygenated blood. The second pathway is "donation after circulatory determination of death," or DCDD, in which organs are removed after a patient has both stopped breathing and been without a pulse for a specified interval (typically between two and five minutes, depending on the protocol). This approach has been most successful for kidney donation, but other organs have been procured in this way as well.

Although most vital organ donors are patients who have been determined to be dead by neurological criteria (brain death), the fastest growing category involves those who have been determined to be dead by circulatory and respiratory criteria. The number of DCDD donors increased from 189 in 2002 to 920 in 2009, and they currently comprise 11% of all vital organ donors (Steinbrook 2007; UNOS 2010). In this chapter we examine critically the determination of death that precedes organ procurement under DCDD protocols. In contrast to our critique of "brain death," the key issue is not the cogency of the criteria for determining death but the application of circulatory and respiratory criteria to the situation of these vital organ donors.

The procurement of organs from DCDD donors actually represents the revitalization of an old practice. Prior to 1968 and the development of the Harvard brain-death criteria, most organs were obtained from patients whose hearts were no longer beating. This approach fell out of favor after the adoption of brain-death criteria, since use of these criteria permitted transplant surgeons to remove vital organs from patients who remained on mechanical ventilation and while their hearts were still beating, allowing the surgeons to remove living organs from a body that was legally dead. Over the past decade, however, the number of brain-dead donors has essentially leveled off at about 5000 donors per year, while the waiting lists for organs have continued to grow. This increasingly unmet need, in combination with the development of improved methods to preserve organs that have been removed from patients after cardiac arrest, has led to renewed interest in DCDD as a source of transplantable organs.

The University of Pittsburgh was the first institution to actively promote DCDD in the early 1990s, and for many years this approach was commonly referred to as the "Pittsburgh Protocol" (DeVita and Snyder 1993; University of Pittsburgh Medical Center 1993). Since then, enthusiasm for DCDD donation has been expressed by the Institute of Medicine in three separate reports, and in 2007 the Joint Commission implemented an accreditation standard that requires all hospitals to develop policies on DCDD (Steinbrook 2007).

DCDD organ donors are typically individuals who have suffered neurological injuries that are not sufficient for them to fulfill brain-death criteria but that are nonetheless severe enough to make them ventilator dependent (although patients who are neurologically intact but ventilator dependent for other reasons, such as neuromuscular disease or spinal cord injury, can also be DCDD candidates). Standard protocols require that these patients or their surrogates have made an independent decision to withdraw life support—based on an assessment of the benefits and harms of continued treatment and in anticipation of the patient's death—before the possibility of organ donation is presented to the family.

If the patient or surrogate consents to the process, then life support is withdrawn in a controlled fashion. Protocols are highly variable. In some centers, for example, the process occurs in the intensive care unit, whereas others require life support to be withdrawn in the operating room. Some require the placement of catheters in the vessels in the groin before the withdrawal of life support in anticipation of flushing the organs immediately after the patient is declared dead. Most require the administration of heparin before the onset of pulselessness, so as to prevent blood clots from forming in the organs before they can be removed.

Once the ventilator is withdrawn, patients are treated with all of the same comfort measures (including the administration of analgesics and sedatives) that they would receive if they were not a potential organ donor. If the patient does not develop pulselessness within 60 minutes, most protocols require that organ procurement efforts be abandoned, since beyond this time frame the organs are thought to have suffered irreversible damage. If the patient does become pulseless within this window, however, then the patient is observed for a short period of time, typically between 2 and 5 minutes (depending on the protocol), to be sure that apnea and the cessation of pulse are considered irreversible (Institute of Medicine 2000). (Whether it is properly deemed irreversible is a basic issue in contention, which we discuss below.) During this interval, known as the "death watch" (DeVita 2001), the family says their final good-byes, and the patient is prepared for surgery. When the interval has passed without evidence of the return of circulatory or respiratory function, the patient is declared dead, and the organs are expeditiously removed (Bernat et al. 2006b). A recently described case report illustrates a common DCDD scenario:

> A 45-year-old man had a sudden headache followed rapidly by unconsciousness. He was taken to a community hospital emergency department where he required intubation and ventilation. Brain CT scan showed a large right hemispheric intracerebral, intraventricular, and subdural hemorrhage with early brain herniation. On urgent transfer to the medical center, he was deeply comatose with a dilated, unreactive right pupil. Following emergency department insertion of an external ventricular drain, he underwent immediate surgical removal of the intraparenchymal and subdural hemorrhage, removal of a ruptured arteriovenous malformation, and hemicraniectomy. Subsequent CT scans showed large infarctions of both temporal lobes and the right occipital lobe.
>
> On the fifth postoperative day, he remained deeply comatose with elevated intracranial pressures in the 50s. Both pupils were unreactive and all brainstem reflexes were absent. He was overbreathing the ventilator. Brain CT scan showed further brain herniation. Given the dismal neurological prognosis, his family requested withdrawal of life-sustaining therapy and consented to organ donation. With his family at the bedside, he was extubated and apnea was observed. Within minutes, he developed pulseless cardiac electrical activity followed within a minute by asystole. After 5 minutes of asystole and apnea, he was declared dead and rushed to the operating room for organ donation. His liver and kidneys were recovered. (Bernat 2010a; Truog and Miller 2010)

A standard assumption in the ethics of organ donation is that donors must be declared dead before the donation of vital organs—the so-called dead donor rule (DDR) (Robertson 1999). Brain-dead organ donors are declared dead on the basis of neurological criteria, whereas DCDD donors are declared dead on the basis of circulatory and respiratory criteria. In Chapter 3 we argued that brain-dead organ donors are not dead owing to the range of biological functioning of the organism as a whole manifested by these individuals. In this chapter we will present arguments showing that DCDD donors are not dead, or at least are not known to be dead, at the time that vital organs are removed because the cessation of circulation is not necessarily irreversible within a very short interval after the absence of breathing and heart beat have been observed.

Professor James Bernat at Dartmouth Medical School has been the major proponent of DCDD in claiming that the donors are dead and that the practice conforms with the DDR. Hence, many of our views will be presented in contrast to his writings on the subject. It is worth noting at the outset, however, that his own views have changed dramatically over the past several years. In 1998, for example, he expressed a view essentially consonant with our own when he wrote:

It takes considerably longer than a few minutes for the brain and other organs to be destroyed from cessation of circulation and lack of oxygen. Moreover, it takes longer than this time for the cessation of heartbeat and breathing to be unequivocally irreversible, a prerequisite for death. As proof of this assertion, if cardiopulmonary resuscitation were performed within a few minutes of cardiorespiratory arrest, it is likely that some of the purportedly "dead" patients could be successfully resuscitated to spontaneous heartbeat and some intact brain function. . . . the brief absence of heartbeat and breathing is highly predictive of death in this context, but at the time the organs are being procured in the Pittsburgh protocol, death has not yet occurred. (Bernat 1998)

We discuss below how Bernat's views have evolved such that he now believes DCDD donors to be dead, and we explain why we think he had it right in the first place.

DCDD AND THE BRAIN

The Uniform Determination of Death Act (UDDA), accepted in all 50 of the United States, reads: "An individual who has sustained either (1) irreversible cessation of circulatory or respiratory functions, or (2) irreversible cessation of all functions of the entire brain, including the brainstem, is dead. A determination of death must be made in accordance with accepted medical standards" (President's Commission 1981).

The wording of the UDDA seems to imply that the Commission was endorsing two separate and independent criteria for the definition of death, one based on neurological functions and the other based on circulatory and respiratory functions. In the report itself, however, the Commission claims otherwise, insisting that it was not proposing a true redefinition of death, but merely providing a refined understanding of a traditional view that sees neurological functions as central to the definition of life and death (President's Commission 1981, 41). Others regard this claim as historical revisionism, arguing that no consensus exists either historically or even in contemporary culture about whether death is fundamentally defined in terms of neurological or circulatory and respiratory functions (Veatch 1992).

Nevertheless, supporters of the concept of brain death have generally endorsed the view that the UDDA describes two different methods for fulfilling a single criterion. Bernat explains: "Although stated separately, the two standards are essentially a single one based on brain functions" (Bernat et al. 2010a). He believes that "The new ventilator technology of thirty years ago that produced the first cases of brain death did not change the definition of death," and that "Future advances in technology will alter the criterion of death but the impact probably will be minor." He foresees future technologies as elucidating "the exact quantity and location of that critical set of brain neurons whose irreversible cessation of functioning are necessary and sufficient for death" (Bernat 1992).

Against this theoretical background, the shift toward declaring death in DCDD protocols on the basis of circulatory and respiratory function is confusing at best. All of the recommendations, guidelines, and consensus documents that have been developed around DCDD have argued that the necessary duration of the interval between the onset of pulselessness and the declaration of death should be based upon data about when the loss of circulatory function can be considered irreversible. Yet if the loss of circulatory function is merely a proxy for determining the loss of neurological function (as supporters of the concept of brain death consistently maintain), then the focus of inquiry and analysis should be on determining the duration of pulselessness that is necessary to ensure that the loss of neurological function is both complete and irreversible.

Perhaps one reason that this question has been ignored is the fact that it probably takes considerably more than 2–5 minutes of pulselessness for neurological function to be completely and irreversibly lost, as Bernat affirms in the quotation above. A classic neurological textbook on the diagnosis of coma confirms this view: "Under clinical circumstances, total ischemic anoxia of the cerebral cortex lasting longer than about 4 minutes starts to kill brain cells, with the neurons of the cerebral cortex and the cerebellum first" and "In man, severe diffuse ischemic anoxia lasting 10 minutes or more begins to destroy the brain" (Plum and Posner 2007; de Groot and Kompanje 2010).

Despite the commonly expressed view that the UDDA should be understood as referring to a single criterion for the determination of death based upon neurological functions, the justifications that have been offered to support the practice of DCDD imply acceptance of dichotomous criteria for determining death, one based on the irreversible loss of neurological functions, and the other based on the irreversible loss of circulatory and respiratory function. In the next section we examine whether the current guidelines for DCDD provide assurance that the loss of circulatory and respiratory functions is irreversible.

AUTORESUSCITATION

Current guidelines assert that DCDD donors should be declared dead after they have been pulseless and apneic for an interval between 2 and 5 minutes. The UDDA states that patients are dead when the loss of their circulatory and respiratory function is irreversible. A key question, therefore, is whether an interval of 2–5 minutes is sufficient to know whether the loss of these functions is irreversible.

In the debate about DCDD, no one has ever maintained that it is impossible to successfully resuscitate patients after they have been pulseless for 5 minutes or more, since many such successful resuscitations have been documented both within hospitals and by paramedics in the field. Rather, supporters of this practice have pointed out that in this context there has been both an appropriate decision to withdraw life support and a "do-not-attempt-resuscitation" DNAR order placed in the medical record. In these circumstances, it would be unethical (and indeed illegal) for the clinicians to attempt resuscitation in the event of cardiac arrest. Given the fact that no attempt will be made to resuscitate the patient, the claim is made that the duration of documented pulselessness need only be long enough to be sure that the heart will not restart spontaneously on its own, a phenomenon known as autoresuscitation.

The data on autoresuscitation in the medical literature are scant and of poor quality. From the information available, a common assumption has been that autoresuscitation does not occur after 65 seconds of pulselessness (DeVita et al. 2000; DeVita 2001). This has been the basis for the recommendation to wait at least 2 minutes after the onset of pulselessness before declaring death (Institute of Medicine 2000).

The medical and social acceptability of the 2-minute limit was recently tested by the cardiac transplantation team at Denver Children's Hospital. Many severe cardiac anomalies present in the newborn period and are incompatible with life without a cardiac transplant. Pediatric heart donors are relatively rare, and the heart is the organ most sensitive to prolonged periods of anoxia. Based upon the data indicating that autoresuscitation does not occur beyond 65 seconds of pulselessness, the Denver physicians therefore adopted a protocol that permitted the declaration of death after only 75 seconds of pulselessness, and reported on the success of three transplants performed under this protocol (organs were procured from one of the patients after 3 minutes, and from the other two after 75 seconds) (Boucek et al. 2008).

More recently, Hornby and colleagues published the most comprehensive review to date on the phenomenon of autoresuscitation. They did not find *any* cases in which autoresuscitation occurred in patients who did not receive cardiopulmonary resuscitation. Indeed, they disqualified the commonly cited case of autoresuscitation that occurred at 65 seconds, noting that since the patient recovered only electrical cardiac activity and not true cardiac pulsation, the case did not qualify as an autoresuscitation event (Hornby et al. 2010). These data are very important, in that they reveal the complete absence of any evidence base for requiring 75 seconds, 2 minutes, 5 minutes, or any other interval for the death watch in the practice of DCDD. Based on the available data, and using the assumption that death can be declared when the heart is no longer able to autoresuscitate, it would appear that death can be declared literally at the moment of asystole, without any death watch. Of course, it is impossible to determine the exact "moment" of pulselessness, since it depends upon waiting some period of time to be sure the last pulsation was indeed the last.

On the other hand, there are good reasons to be cautious about any attempt to establish an evidence base concerning the phenomenon of autoresuscitation. As Shewmon has described, statistical considerations reveal the difficulty of proving that events will not happen (Shewmon 1987). Consider, for example a study showing the absence of autoresuscitation in N consecutive dying patients. Statistically, the risk of autoresuscitation occurring in the next patient is approximately $1/(N + 2)$, and the chance of at least one episode of autoresuscitation occurring among the next $(N + 1)$ patients who meet the criterion is around 50%. Hence a high-quality case series involving as many as 100 or even 1000 patients (far larger than anything currently available) would still leave a non-negligible level of uncertainty regarding the outcome in the next patient, particularly around something as critical as the diagnosis of death. As Shewmon clearly observes, this does not mean that death cannot be diagnosed on the basis of a criterion like pulselessness, but rather that the validation of such criteria by empirical methods is subject to a degree of uncertainty that would likely be unacceptable for determining the difference between states as important as life and death. Although the existence of a criterion such as pulselessness would be obvious at the extremes (such as after the onset of putrefaction and decay), criteria based on findings such as these would not be useful for the purpose of declaring death in the context of organ transplantation. In other words, these statistical considerations show that attempts to use empirical methods to establish the diagnosis of death after only several minutes of pulselessness are unlikely to be convincing.

DCDD AND IRREVERSIBILITY

Although the notion that irreversibility can be defined in terms of the possibility of autoresuscitation has been prevalent in the DCDD literature for years, the report of the successful heart transplants in Denver kindled a burst of skepticism about this approach to defining death. In response to the report, several commentators made the rather obvious but nevertheless incisive observation that if a donor's death is pronounced on the basis of the irreversible loss of cardiac function, and then the heart is successfully transplanted and functions in the chest of another, then the loss of cardiac function could not have been *irreversible*, at least in any common sense understanding of the term (Truog and Miller 2008; Veatch 2008). As Veatch put it: "it would simply not be possible to perform successful heart transplantation in a manner consistent with the dead donor rule after death pronounced on the basis of cardiac criteria" (Veatch 2008).

Indeed, some transplant centers have been reluctant to perform cardiac transplantation from DCDD donors, precisely because they have not wanted to stir debate about whether the donors were really dead. But Marquis has noted that the problem runs even deeper than this. If we are concerned that the actual transplantation of a heart from a DCDD donor would be in violation of the DDR, then it would also be the case that if the heart *could have been* transplanted (and functioned effectively), then the DDR would also be violated, even if only noncardiac organs were actually transplanted, since vital organs would have been removed before the cessation of cardiac function was irreversible (Marquis 2010). Since the Denver team reported a successful heart transplant from a patient after 3 minutes of pulselessness, the validity of the 2-minute rule used by many transplant centers is thereby called into question.

Bernat has responded to these critiques by arguing that they have mistakenly focused upon the function of the heart, rather than the circulation more generally (Bernat et al. 2010a). He points out that the UDDA refers to "circulatory," not "cardiac" function, and therefore has lobbied in favor of changing the name of the practice from "donation after cardiac death" (DCD) to "donation after circulatory determination of death" (DCDD). Although we see nothing wrong with this clarification of the terminology (and adopt his recommendation in this book), we do not think that this linguistic refinement does anything to refute the fundamental objection. If the loss of cardiac function in these donors was not irreversible, then there is no reason to think that the loss of circulatory function was irreversible either, at least up until the time at which the heart is removed from the donor's body for transplantation.

Veatch has also recently explored whether we could declare irreversibility in the body of the donor while not implying that the condition must be irreversible in the body of the recipient. He wrote, "One work around to this problem—that is, that patients suffering cardiac arrests that can and will be reversed are not dead—would be to further amend the definition of death law to hold that heart irreversibility applies only while the heart is still in the original patient's body. . . However, this seems strangely like gerrymandering our definition" (Veatch 2010). We agree.

DCDD AND INTENTIONS

As noted above, the use of autoresuscitation data in the development of DCDD protocols depends upon the idea that a function can be regarded as irreversibly lost when it would be wrong to attempt to restore the function and when the function cannot restart on its own. Because DCDD donors must have a DNAR order in place before the withdrawal of life support, and because autoresuscitation apparently does not occur in this setting, by this argument their circulatory function has irreversibly ceased. This argument is flawed, we believe, because it makes determinations of life and death dependent upon the intentions and actions of others.

The difference between life and death is a biological and an ontological distinction; it is about two different "states of the world." But under the current formulation, this fundamental distinction becomes dependent upon the intentions and actions of those surrounding the patient at the time of death. Consider, for example, the following thought experiment:

Case 1: An otherwise healthy young athlete is involved in a severe automobile accident, leaving him with devastating brain injury but not brain death. He is taken to the operating room for DCDD organ donation, becomes pulseless shortly after the withdrawal of life support, and remains pulseless for 2 minutes. Is he dead?

Case 2: An otherwise healthy young athlete collapses in pulseless V-fib arrest while playing basketball. No one initiates CPR. After 2 minutes paramedics arrive. Is he already dead?

Using the current reasoning about DCDD, and assuming that it would be appropriate for the paramedics to initiate cardiopulmonary resuscitation (CPR) in Case 2, the young man is dead in Case 1 but not dead (or at least not known to be dead) in Case 2. The only difference relevant to a determination of death between these cases is whether those who are present intend to initiate CPR. If death is a natural fact or state of the world that exists independent of our thoughts, opinions, and intentions, then the status of these two individuals as dead or alive should be treated the same.

Case 3: Consider a variation of Case 1 where the young man's parents are present during the withdrawal of life support and when death is declared after 2 minutes of pulselessness. But imagine that in their overwhelming grief they suddenly change their minds, and demand that rescuscitation be attempted. Imagine that the clinicians comply and are successful (a reasonable possibility). Has the patient been raised from the dead?

As Bernat has correctly observed, "Because no mortal can return from being dead, any resuscitation or recovery must have been from a state of dying but not from death" (Bernat 2006b). Following this reasoning, it would seem that this patient was not in fact dead, but only dying, at the time that death was declared. Brock has succinctly summed up the problem with treating the cessation of circulation as irreversible and the donor as dead in the context of DCDD protocols: "The common sense understanding of the irreversibility of death is that it is not *possible* to restore the life or life functions of the individual, not that they will not in fact be restored only because no attempt will be made to do so" (Brock 1999, 298).

DCDD AND PERMANENCE

Bernat has acknowledged that the UDDA refers to the "irreversible" loss of circulatory function, and that since the term irreversible means that "the function cannot be restored by any known technology" (Bernat et al. 2010), it may appear that DCDD donors are not really dead. He argues that this interpretation would not be correct, however. He refers back to the report of the President's Commission, *Defining Death*, citing it as the principal piece of legislative history available, and notes that in this document the term "irreversible" is used interchangeably with the term "permanent." He explains that the terms differ in that "a 'permanent' cessation of function means that the function will not be restored because it will neither return spontaneously, nor will return as a result of medical intervention because resuscitation efforts will not be attempted" (Bernat et al. 2010). With regard to DCDD donors, permanence "represents an earlier stage of an inevitable process that rapidly and with complete certainty yields irreversibility." "Permanence," he concludes, "is the absolute prognosis of irreversibility" (Bernat 2006b).

Based on this analysis, is Bernat correct that "permanent cessation serves as a valid stand-in for irreversible cessation" (Bernat et al. 2010)? In the context of DCDD, the implication is that since permanence is 100% predictive of irreversibility, when patients meet the criteria for permanence, they can be treated as if they meet the criteria for irreversibility. This stance unfortunately conflates a *prognosis* of imminent death with a *diagnosis* of death. Even if it is true that permanence infallibly predicts irreversibility, it does not follow that when the cessation of circulation is permanent, the patient is already dead (as distinct from about to be dead). Consider some of the very implausible implications of this line of reasoning:

> *Case 4: A young man has been a quadriplegic for several years following a diving accident which transected his upper cervical spinal cord. He is unable to generate any breathing movements, and is completely dependent upon mechanical ventilation. After long consideration, he requests that his ventilator be withdrawn, knowing that he will die. If his ventilator is withdrawn, his prognosis for death is 100%.*
>
> *Case 5: A young man with acute severe cardiomyopathy is being supported with extracorporeal membrane oxygenation (ECMO), a form of cardiopulmonary bypass. Echocardiograms show that he has no cardiac function (his heart is at standstill). He has refused the option of being listed for a heart transplant, and has requested that ECMO be discontinued, knowing that he will die. If ECMO is withdrawn, his prognosis for death is 100%.*

At the moment of ventilator or ECMO withdrawal, both of these patients meet Bernat's criterion for the permanent loss of circulatory function, since both are 100% certain to quickly fulfill the criteria for the irreversible loss of circulatory function. Yet certainly no one would argue that at the moment of ventilator or ECMO withdrawal either of these patients is already dead. In particular, it would clearly be wrong to initiate organ procurement at this moment without providing them with an anesthetic.

To push the point even further, if we agree with Bernat that the intentions of others can play a role in determining death, then it would appear that both of these patients could be declared dead even before withdrawal of the ventilator or ECMO, since acting upon this intention is also 100% predictive of imminently fulfilling the criteria for the irreversible loss of circulatory function. Although it may be ethically acceptable to permit both of these patients to donate vital organs before or after the withdrawal of life support (with an anesthetic if necessary), as we argue in Chapter 6, the reason it may be ethical cannot be because they are already dead.

Finally, treating permanence as a valid indicator of irreversibility fails to reflect the critical difference in the logic of these two concepts. As Marquis observes, "A condition is permanent if the condition is never actually reversed. A condition is irreversible if the condition never *could* be reversed. In short, irreversibility entails permanence; permanence does not entail irreversibility.

Therefore, given the plain meaning of the terms, the permanence of the cessation of circulatory function in DCD donors does not entail its irreversibility" (Marquis 2010, 26). Under DCDD protocols it is true that cessation of circulation following ventilator withdrawal will not be reversed, given the decision not to attempt resuscitation. It therefore is permanent. But the realistic possibility that it could be reversed if resuscitation were attempted means that the cessation of circulation is not known to be irreversible; hence the donor is not known to be dead at the time that vital organs are procured.

ACCEPTED MEDICAL PRACTICE

In his most recent writings, Bernat seems to acknowledge the force of the objections raised above, and has fallen back on defending permanence as a "valid stand-in" irreversibility on the authority of "accepted medical practice." In a statement with several colleagues, he declares:

> We acknowledge that, from a purely ontological perspective, the human being is not dead until the cessation of brain functions or of circulation and respiration is irreversible. But. . . medical practice standards that have been unquestionably accepted by physicians and society permit physicians to declare death at the moment that cessation of circulation and respiration can be shown to be permanent. Thus, death determination in donation after circulatory determination of death donors and other patients is fundamentally a medical practice issue and not primarily a moral or ontological issue. (Bernat et al. 2010)

In defending this view, he offers three examples for consideration, all based on the observation that in a variety of end-of-life scenarios, physicians commonly declare patients to be dead at the time that their heart stops beating, prior to the time when the physicians could know that the loss of circulatory function has become irreversible (Bernat 2006b, 2010b; Bernat et al. 2010).

We agree that Bernat has accurately described "accepted medical practice" in the context of end-of-life care that does not involve organ donation. But we believe this observation is irrelevant in situations in which following the dead donor rule requires us to know whether the patient is merely dying or already dead. In this context, as in many areas of medicine, the accuracy that is required of our assessments depends upon the consequences of our assessments being wrong.

For example, a physician who needs to be absolutely certain that a patient is well hydrated before giving a nephrotoxic drug will use different criteria for assessment than if he or she is merely interested in knowing if the patient is in good fluid balance outside of a potentially toxic insult. If a physician is about to amputate a limb for what is believed to be a local malignancy, he or she will use more precise criteria to rule out metastatic disease than if amputation is not a feasible therapeutic option. In other words, the criteria physicians use to establish the presence or absence of a clinical condition are context dependent. We cannot say that because the use of certain criteria are "accepted medical practice" in many common end-of-life situations this is proof that they are adequate in other end-of-life contexts, such as DCDD, where (assuming the necessity of the DDR) it is crucial to be certain whether the patient is still dying or already dead.

In Napoleon's empire, physicians were prohibited from declaring death until they had performed a death watch for 24 hours (Pernick 1988). In today's hospitals, we commonly declare death at the moment of asystole, confident that nothing consequential will happen to the patient over the next several minutes, and that the routine flow of hospital activity will provide an adequate death watch to ensure that the criteria for irreversibility are satisfied. But when the few minutes following the onset of asystole may involve lethal actions such as the removal of vital organs, the methods of assessment must be correspondingly more precise. Moreover, *if* the DDR is an inviolate principle of vital organ donation, then the difference between "dying" and "dead" becomes very important. Even a very slim chance of a false positive makes a difference. If the patient is in fact not dead or not known to be dead at the time of the declaration of death, then the DDR has been violated.

DCDD AND ECMO

Extracorporeal membrane oxygenation (ECMO) is a form of cardiopulmonary bypass that is used in intensive care units to provide life support for patients with severe respiratory or cardiac failure. Typically, large cannulas (plastic tubes) are passed through skin incisions into the large arteries and veins of the body. Venous blood is drained out of the heart, pumped through a membrane oxygenator (artificial lung), and then returned to the aorta. The external pump replaces cardiac function; the membrane oxygenator replaces respiratory function. Patients on ECMO must be anticoagulated with heparin to prevent clotting of the circuit. The technology is often used for up to several weeks; the duration is not limited by the technology itself, but by associated complications such as bleeding and infection.

Under the leadership of Dr. Robert Bartlett, the University of Michigan has been at the forefront in the continued development of ECMO technology. Michigan is one of a few centers that have explored the use of ECMO in improving the feasibility and efficiency of DCDD (which we will refer to as E-DCDD). In one approach, DCDD candidates have ECMO cannulas placed in the femoral artery and vein in their groin before the withdrawal of life support. After the requisite 5 minutes of pulselessness, the ECMO machine is turned on. This "reanimates" the organs that are now once again being perfused with warm oxygenated blood.

Without modification of the ECMO circuit, all of the organs of the body, including the brain, would be reanimated. To prevent cerebral resuscitation, balloon-tipped catheters are placed and inflated in certain vessels to block the flow of blood. If the balloon is placed in the distal aorta, the circulation of blood is restricted to those organs that are below the diaphragm (kidneys, liver, pancreas, intestine). If balloons are placed in the four major arteries that supply the brain, then the thoracic organs (heart and lungs) can be perfused as well. Another variation that has been proposed that would not involve the use of balloon catheters would be to increase the death watch to 10 minutes or more before perfusing the entire body, on the assumption that after this much time the patient would be brain dead and it would be impossible to resuscitate the brain.

Once the patient is on ECMO, there is no rush to remove the organs. In traditional DCDD, once the 2–5 minute death watch is over, the organs must be removed as soon as possible, precluding the family from spending time with and grieving over their deceased loved one. For patients who are on ECMO, however, the family can spend as much time as they want with the body before the patient is transported to the operating room on ECMO for organ recovery (Gravel et al. 2004).

This approach seems to be technically very successful. As of early 2009, the Michigan program had performed successful E-DCDD donations from 48 patients, with a 33% increase in the donor pool (Magliocca et al. 2005; Bartlett 2009). In addition, the quality of the organs obtained in this way seems to be better than with traditional DCDD, with rates of organ function comparable to that obtained from brain-dead donors (Magliocca et al. 2005). The use of ECMO also appears to make the duration of pulselessness less critical for organ viability. Their experimental work suggests that organs resuscitated with ECMO can be functional even after 10 minutes or more of pulselessness.

To date, the University of Michigan has not used E-DCDD to procure hearts for transplantation, although they believe this may be technically feasible. In fact, in those cases in which the thoracic organs are perfused, they have deliberately added lidocaine to the perfusate, a drug that specifically affects electrical conductance in the heart and prevents the heart from beginning to beat again. This is done to avoid the type of controversy generated by the Denver protocol over whether the donors are really dead.

In a recent consensus statement, Bernat and colleagues were critical of E-DCDD protocols, describing them as "disturbingly invasive." By deliberately seeking to reanimate the body after the declaration of death, they wonder if these protocols serve "only to satisfy the letter of the UDDA while violating its spirit." They were particularly concerned that the premortem placement of ECMO cannulas would interfere with the quality of palliative care for the patient and family, and yet the E-DCDD protocols do have the advantage of allowing the family to be with the patient for an unlimited period of time after death, a distinct advantage over the requirements of traditional DCDD. In sum, the authors of this consensus statement concluded that these protocols are "undesirable because they are disproportionately invasive and may jeopardize the trustworthiness of the donation process" (Bernat et al. 2010).

We share many of these concerns about the invasiveness of this approach, but suggest that these developments are a predictable consequence of the perceived need to enforce the ethical mandate of the DDR without persuasive reasons for believing that it represents a necessary ethical commitment. These developments further indicate that the DDR is being honored "in the breach," with the development of new approaches and technologies that achieve an "end-run" around the principle whenever feasible. Indeed, it is not difficult to imagine an extension of the current approach that would involve surgically exposing and isolating transplantable organs before the withdrawal of life support, using an anesthetic to ensure the comfort of the patient. Using this technique, organs could be immediately preserved and procured the moment that death was pronounced. Although perhaps upsetting to consider, there is currently nothing in the ethics of DCDD that would rule out this approach, and it would be fully consistent with the DDR.

DCDD AND THE DDR

In concluding this chapter, we must acknowledge that Bernat's attempts to justify the practice of DCDD over the past decade have been motivated by his firmly held belief that any deviation from our current allegiance to the DDR would undermine the trust of the public in the transplantation enterprise, perhaps to the point of jeopardizing our ability to procure organs and save lives. But these efforts, which seek to link determinations of life and death to the intentions of others, or that promote the concept of permanence as a valid proxy for irreversibility, are ultimately flawed attempts to retrofit traditional ethical principles to emerging practice. In some of his writings, Bernat seems to acknowledge the need to bend our principles in order to achieve a greater good, as when he wrote that "if DCD does violate the dead donor rule, it comprises a justified exception," that society will "tolerate knowing that patients are serving as vital organ donors before they are unequivocally dead," and that "most DCD patients will not care if they are declared dead earlier in a process that quickly and inevitably achieves irreversibility, because they wish to donate, and the difference to them is utterly inconsequential" (Bernat 2006b). We agree with Bernat on all of these points, but we believe that this practice can be better defended and justified than by contorted and unsuccessful attempts to make it comply with the DDR.

In sum, the de facto violation of the DDR in current practices of organ donation suggests that we should shift the focus of ethical inquiry from when is it legitimate to determine that an organ donor is dead to when is it legitimate to procure vital organs. The critical issue is not whether the patient-donor is already dead, in order to satisfy the DDR, but whether valid decisions have been made to bring about death of the patient by stopping life-sustaining treatments and to donate organs. If such valid decisions have been made, no harm or wrong is done by procuring vital organs prior to death, for the patient will be dead in a short interval of time as a result of stopping life support regardless of whether organs are procured. The absence of harm plus appropriate consent legitimates vital organ donation. The DDR does no genuine moral work in current practices of vital organs donation because "brain-dead" donors remain alive and donors under DCDD protocols are not known to be dead at the time organs are procured. We should be working toward honestly facing the fact that currently we are procuring vital organs from patients who are not known to be dead and that it is ethically legitimate and desirable to do so. In Chapter 6, we develop these ideas in detail.

6

Vital Organ Donation without the Dead Donor Rule

The established ethical framework for the transplantation of vital organs requires that donors are determined to be dead prior to organ procurement. This is known as the dead donor rule (DDR). However, Albert Jonsen noted that "it is not quite correct to say that an organ can be removed from a dead person and transplanted to a living person. The removed organ must be viable, in the sense that it retains those biological properties that will enable it to function within the recipient. Thus, the body of the donor must still have some sort of vitality at the time of removal" (Jonsen 1989, 235). How can a dead body retain "some sort of vitality"? Gary Greenberg posed this conundrum more sharply in a *New Yorker* article, provocatively titled, "As Good as Dead" (Greenberg 2001). He noted that "[b]y the nineteen-sixties, as doctors began to perfect techniques for transplanting livers and hearts, the medical establishment faced a paradox: the need for both a living body and a dead donor." We have argued in previous chapters that our current practices of vital organ donation, although deemed to be consistent with the DDR, in fact violate it. Brain-dead donors, though drastically compromised neurologically, remain fully alive, while being maintained on life support. Donors under donation after circulatory determination of death (DCDD) protocols are not known to be dead, based on the irreversible cessation of circulatory functioning, when organs are procured a very short interval after asystole. In other words, in view of the biological conception of death adopted in standard medical practice, there is no satisfactory resolution of the paradox.

If this understanding of our current practices is true, then conventional medical ethics would dictate that vital organ donation should cease, because doctors are prohibited from extracting vital organs from living donors and are forbidden to intentionally cause the death of patients. We believe that very few ethicists, clinicians, and members of the public would be prepared to endorse this conclusion. For this would put a stop to life-saving transplantation of hearts, lungs, and livers, and would curtail life-enhancing transplantation of kidneys, which permit patients to be free of dialysis. Currently, over 108,000 patients are on the waiting list in the United States for donor organs (Stein 2010). Accordingly, if we are to continue to transplant vital organs, it is necessary to construct a sound ethical justification for vital organ donation that does not rely on the DDR. This requires honestly facing the fact that vital organs are being procured from still-living patients, rather than dead bodies, and showing that doing so is ethical. As a preliminary step in this search for ethical justification, it will be useful to probe the ethical considerations thought to underlie the DDR.

THE DEAD DONOR RULE

The DDR has the status of a moral axiom governing the practice of vital organ donation (Robertson 1999). To many it appears self-evident, and we are not aware of any systematic efforts to justify this moral rule. A basic principle underlying the DDR is that doctors must not kill their patients, which is a specification of a more general ethical prohibition of intentional killing of innocent persons. Additionally, the DDR is seen as a protection against exploitation. No person should be sacrificed and treated merely as a means for obtaining vital organs to save the lives of others. We have addressed the first principle regarding medical killing in Chapters 1 and 2. We argued that the traditional principle of medical ethics that doctors must not kill must be abandoned in the context of patient care with respect to end-of-life decisions, because the justified routine practice of withdrawing life-sustaining treatment (LST) causes the deaths of patients. Additionally, we argued that an ethical bright line between withdrawing LST and active euthanasia by lethal injection, whereby the former is justifiable, because it allows patients to die, but the latter is always wrong, because it kills patients, cannot withstand critical scrutiny. In this chapter we argue that current practices of transplantation are ethically justified despite the fact that they involve procuring vital organs from donors who are not dead (or not known to be dead), thereby contravening the DDR. Although the DDR must be abandoned, vital organ transplantation can be performed without exploitatively sacrificing vulnerable patients to save the lives of others. In other words, a significant part of the ethical rationale supporting the DDR can be retained even though the rule itself must be abandoned if we are to be forthright in justifying transplantation of vital organs.

AN ALTERNATIVE ETHICAL FRAMEWORK:
ABSENCE OF HARM AND CONSENT

The ethics of withdrawing LST, recognizing that this causes death, underlies the justification for vital organ donation from still-living patients. First, it demonstrates that causing death in medicine is not necessarily wrong. More importantly, making vital organ donation conditional on and subsequent in time to prior valid decisions to withdraw LST places an important constraint on procuring vital organs from still-living patients. This ethical constraint protects vulnerable patients from harm and exploitation and preserves the professional integrity of clinicians.

The basic justificatory consideration is that when patients have a prior valid plan in place to withdraw LST and proper consent has been obtained for organ donation, they are not harmed or wronged by procuring vital organs while they are still alive. In this context, no harm (or wrong) is done to the patient-donor by procuring vital organs prior to a death-causing treatment withdrawal, provided that any potential for suffering from the procurement procedure is neutralized by adequate anesthesia. Harms are setbacks to a person's or being's interests (Feinberg 1984; Beauchamp and Childress 2009). Patients whose organs are donated in the context of a prior planned withdrawal of LST are not harmed because they have no interests that are set back by procurement of organs before treatment is withdrawn. Specifically, and most importantly, the patient's interest in continued living is not set back by the decision to donate organs because an independent prior decision has been made to stop life support. The patient will die soon in any case, owing to the decision to withdraw LST. In other words, at the time that the decision to withdraw LST is implemented, the patient no longer has any need for vital organs, which can be made available for life-saving transplantation without harming or wronging the donor. (A slight qualification to this claim that no patient-donor is harmed by vital organ procurement under our ethical framework is discussed below in the context of responding to an objection relating to the uncertainty about whether withdrawing LST will cause death in particular cases.)

The death-causing plan to stop LST opens the door to the legitimacy of procuring vital organs from the still-living patient prior to treatment withdrawal. When a patient or surrogate makes a valid decision to withdraw LST, the patient is on a planned trajectory with death as the imminent outcome following treatment withdrawal. Extracting vital organs before the withdrawal does not change this trajectory or infringe on the interests of patients who will die either as the outcome of organ donation or the joint process of organ procurement and treatment withdrawal. Absent the decision to donate vital organs, these patients would have died by stopping LST.

Consider two hospitalized patients A and B, both with the same medical condition and both receiving mechanical ventilation. Surrogate decision makers for A and B decide to stop treatment based on the patients' prior expressed preferences in light of the prognosis of almost no chance of being weaned off the ventilator and being able to return home. In the case of B, but not A, the subsequent decision is made to donate his heart, lungs, and kidneys prior to stopping life support. A dies within a short period of time after stopping the ventilator; B dies in the process of procuring vital organs. We submit that B is not harmed by vital organ donation, though still living at the time that the operation to procure organs is initiated, and is no worse off than A.

Assuming that withdrawing LST would cause the death of the patient, when vital organ donation is conditional on a prior plan of treatment withdrawal, no one is made dead by the process of procuring vital organs (or the combination of this process and the treatment withdrawal) who would not otherwise be made dead by withdrawing LST. In other words, these patients have a life-ending plan of care, which is not changed detrimentally to their interest by procuring vital organs provided they are free of suffering during the process and valid consent is given for the donation. To repeat, making organ donation conditional on and subsequent to a prior valid decision to withdraw LST entails that no harm or wrong comes to the still-living donor by procuring organs prior to stopping treatment. The prior plan to withdraw LST creates the moral possibility for a life-saving donation of vital organs to another patient. The ethical procurement of vital organs does not require adherence to the DDR.

To the extent possible, the prior decision to withdraw LST must be insulated from the decision to donate vital organs. Otherwise, the former decision may be made for the sake of the latter, and it becomes possible that the vulnerable patient might be sacrificed to save the lives of others. Transplant clinicians and those who are caring for potential organ recipients should play no role in the decision to stop life support. Ethics consultation may be desirable to ensure that the prior decision to withdraw LST is being made on appropriate grounds, with respect to the preferences of the patient and the patient's best interests, and independently of the decision to donate organs.

Making the decision to donate vital organs conditional on the prior decision to withdraw LST is critical to the claim that no interests of the patient-donor are set back by procuring vital organs. Consider the case of a patient with high-level cervical quadriplegia who decides to withdraw mechanical ventilation because he judges that his life is no longer worth living. Having made that fateful decision, he also wishes to donate his organs. Currently, this is possible under DCDD protocols. We contend, however, that it is ethically justifiable for the organs to be procured *prior* to stopping LST. The fact that this would violate the DDR does not preclude ethical justification; moreover, as we argued in Chapter 5, DCDD protocols currently also violate the DDR. The decision to stop LST for a patient who could live many more years with a quality of life that most patients with this condition find satisfactory is controversial (Miller 2009a). Clearly, it is not the case that patients with this condition have no interests that would be set back by stopping life support and procuring their organs for transplantation. However, having made the decision to die by stopping mechanical ventilation, this patient now has no basic interests that are set back by procuring vital organs prior to stopping treatment. To be sure, the interest in a peaceful and dignified death might be compromised to some extent by requiring that the patient's last moments are spent in the operating room of a hospital rather than at home with the aid of hospice. But the patient has freely decided to donate organs and thus forgo what might otherwise be the preferred way to die in order to save the lives of others. Importantly, no compromise in comfort during the process would be needed to achieve the joint preferences of stopping LST and donating organs.

Beyond the absence of harm, vital organ donation is justified by a double process of consent: first, as a necessary prior condition, there must be valid consent to withdraw LST, which is equivalent to a valid refusal of treatment; second, valid consent is provided to donate organs. The requirement of valid consents for stopping treatment and donating organs means that the patient-donors are not wronged, despite the fact that they are not dead prior to procuring vital organs. In most cases, these contemporaneous dual consents will be provided by surrogates authorizing treatment withdrawal and organ donation on behalf of the incapacitated patient, though these decisions should to the extent possible be based on advance directives or prior statements of preferences by the patient. Insofar as it is justifiable to cause the patient's death by withdrawing LST, based on a valid refusal of continued life support, it is also thereby justifiable to extract vital organs prior to stopping LST when doing so is validly authorized.

It is important to recognize that consent for vital organ donation under the ethical framework that we advocate differs from the current practice of informed consent for organ donation, which is predicated on the assumption that these donors are dead. Prospective consent of donors or contemporaneous consent of surrogates would need to be based on recognition that the donor diagnosed as "brain dead" remains alive and will die as the result of the process of organ procurement and stopping LST. Likewise, consent for vital organ donation for patients on life support who are not "brain dead" would involve authorizing organ procurement prior to stopping LST. Would it be harder to obtain consent for vital organ donation from such patients who are recognized as still living?

This depends on attitudes of the public toward vital organ donation when donors are recognized as still living though soon to be dead owing to a valid decision to withdraw LST, which we discuss below.

In the next section we expand and bolster this ethical framework by considering and replying to a series of objections. In the course of this discussion, we address the issue of professional integrity of clinicians involved in procuring vital organs, which is a necessary component of a comprehensive justification of vital organ donation without the DDR.

OBJECTIONS AND REPLIES

Differences between Withdrawing Treatment and Lethal Organ Procurement

Against this ethical framework, it may be objected that extracting vital organs from a still-living patient necessarily causes death, whereas stopping life support does not. Is the element of uncertainty about causing death by withdrawing LST ethically relevant in a way that permits this practice but makes it categorically wrong to procure vital organs from living donors? This objection deserves attention, but it should be noted that its force is limited to organ donors on life support who are not "brain dead." We know with certainty that there is no prospect for continued life for "brain-dead" donors once mechanical ventilation is stopped. Such absolute certainty is not possible, however, for other donors on life support, since some might be able to survive withdrawal of mechanical ventilation, as in the case of Karen Quinlan discussed in Chapter 1. Withdrawing LST generally causes death, but it does not cause death in all circumstances. Our justification of vital organ donation makes this conditional on a prior plan to withdraw LST, on the assumption that treatment withdrawal is sufficient to cause death. If, in fact, the patient would not have died following the withdrawal of LST, then the process of organ donation would itself lead to the death of a patient who would not otherwise have died. We believe that this concern can be addressed by an examination of our current approach to palliative care at the end of life.

Withdrawal of LST occurs in two very different contexts. In one typical scenario, the clinicians and surrogate may choose to withdraw treatments such as mechanical ventilation, uncertain of whether the patient may be able to survive without support, but with a plan not to reinstitute the treatment if the patient cannot sustain unassisted respiration. Under these circumstances, opioids and any other respiratory depressants are avoided, at least until the clinical trajectory of the patient becomes better defined. Patients in this category, undergoing a trial to determine if they can survive without life support, would not be acceptable candidates for vital organ donation.

In the other and more common context, LST such as mechanical ventilation is withdrawn in the belief that the patient will not be able to sustain unassisted respiration. In these cases, no attempt is made to avoid opioids and other comfort medications that depress respiration, since doing so would subject the patient to unnecessary pain and suffering. Indeed, in such cases standard palliative care involves premedicating patients with opioids and other sedatives before ventilator withdrawal, with additional medications added following withdrawal, titrated to the patient's response and degree of comfort (Truog et al. 2001, 2008). This approach necessarily means that some patients may succumb to respiratory failure and death who might have survived if they had not been treated for their shortness of breath and sense of suffocation. The proportion of such patients is not known, but is probably only a very small fraction of those who have LST withdrawn. Accordingly, there is an inherent trade-off built into our standard approach to end-of-life care: rather than refrain from the use of any respiratory depressants with the consequent suffering of many who would die regardless, we accept that some patients who might have survived treatment withdrawal for some period of time actually have their deaths hastened as a result of the medications clinicians administer.

In this context, we argue that our proposed justification of vital organ donation is compatible with the current approach to end-of-life care. It is true that because of an imperfect ability to prognosticate death after withdrawal of LST, some patients will die who might otherwise have continued to live. In all cases, however, this will occur in circumstances in which the physicians believe that the patient is very unlikely to survive withdrawal of LST and when the patient's surrogate is expecting and is prepared for the patient's death, believing that this outcome is better for the patient than continued, burdensome, life support. Again, there is a trade-off—in the first case between a small number of survivors versus the comfort of all patients who have LST withdrawn, and under our proposal between these potential survivors and the possibility of organ donation, with all of its benefits for the recipients as well as for honoring the donation preferences of the donor. In any case, when there has been a justifiable prior decision to stop LST, it is also justifiable to cause the patient's death by this act. The element of uncertainty in causation is not ethically relevant to the justification of withdrawing life support. Nor does it obviate the basic ethical premise that no harm or wrong is done to the patient-donor when procuring vital organs precedes treatment withdrawal, especially in the context of valid consent.

The possibility that the patient following withdrawing LST might have recovered to a satisfactory quality of life, and thus would have been harmed by the death-causing act of procuring vital organs, is too remote to undermine this justificatory framework for vital organ donation. This possibility, however, indicates the need, for the sake of exactitude, to qualify our key claim that no interests of patient-donors are set back by vital organ donation under our justificatory conditions. For those who are on life support but not "brain dead" there is a vanishingly small, but not zero, chance that even though sedated prior to treatment withdrawal (in the absence of vital organ procurement), they would recover to a satisfactory quality of life. These, and only these, patients could be harmed by death-causing vital organ procurement prior to treatment withdrawal. (When we repeat the claim that patient-donors are not harmed by vital organ procurement, this qualification will be assumed.) Furthermore, valid consent to the conjunction of withdrawing LST and vital organ donation presupposes comprehension of the certainty that the donor will die. When such consent is obtained, no wrong is done to the donor by causing death in this way. No such qualification about harm is needed for those organ donors who are "brain dead." If properly diagnosed, these patients cannot survive the withdrawal of mechanical ventilation.

Nonetheless, equating the death-causing act of procuring vital organs with that of withdrawing LST will be challenged. Isn't cutting out the heart from a still-living patient a very different act from stopping the ventilator, notwithstanding the fact that both acts cause death? It is different and feels different. However, the descriptive and psychological differences do not entail that whereas the latter is justifiable the former is not. Consider first the case of organ donation from "brain-dead" donors. This involves procuring vital organs while the donor remains on the ventilator and is receiving other life-support measures. This practice currently is understood as operating on a dead body and is justified only if the body is dead. But we have argued that patients diagnosed as satisfying the clinical criteria for "brain death" remain alive. The declaration of death that precedes organ procurement is based on a fiction in light of the established biological definition of death. When the fiction is exposed, if we continue to hold that vital organ donation from those diagnosed as "brain dead" is justifiable, it cannot be based on the premise that the donor is already dead at the time that organs are procured.

Some might object that acknowledging, as a matter of fact, that the "brain dead" remain alive makes all the difference in the world regarding the ethics of vital organ donation. Taking vital organs from a corpse is one thing; taking them from a living human being, regardless of how compromised, is certainly another. Of course, it is different, but is this difference ethically decisive, such that the former but not the latter is permitted? This is not a matter on which we can expect any universal consensus, as some are committed to a strict stance on the sanctity of human life, such that recognizing the still-living status of "brain-dead" patients suffices to prohibit vital organ donation. But, to be consistent, it should also prohibit stopping life support, given that withdrawing LST causes death. Few will find this position morally palatable. Moreover, although "brain death" does not constitute death, most people are likely to see the patient's condition as making the patient "as good as dead." (Below we discuss in some detail the concept of being "as good as dead.") Although merely vegetative life can be maintained by technological measures, these patients remain permanently unconscious, with absolutely no prospect of regaining sentience. Additionally, because these patients lack any capacity for experience, owing to profound brain damage and the absence of any responsiveness to stimuli indicative of sensory awareness, they have no interests that would be impaired by procuring vital organs while being maintained temporarily on life support. Hence, the justification of vital organ donation from these patients, conditional on a prior plan to withdraw life support, is augmented by consideration of the lack of any quality of life that is the lot of these most unfortunate patients. The prior valid decision to stop life support, which is sufficient to cause death, makes it legitimate to procure vital organs beforehand.

When "brain-dead" vital organ donors are recognized as still living, and procurement of organs is justified by the absence of harm and consent, the only practical change in the sequence of events that procures their organs for transplantation is the absence of a prior declaration of death. In contrast, the situation of patients currently donating organs under DCDD protocols would be treated differently under our ethical framework. The ethical justification of vital organ donation without the DDR, conditional on a prior valid decision to withdraw LST, obviates the need to undergo the elaborate orchestration of DCDD protocols ostensibly aimed at ensuring that the donor is dead on the basis of circulatory criteria before retrieving organs. In fact, however, such donors are not known to be dead within a few minutes after their hearts stop beating: if resuscitative measures could be successful in restoring circulation, then cessation of circulation is not irreversible and the patient would not be dead. In view of the planned, death-causing withdrawal of life support, which currently precedes procurement of organs under these DCDD protocols, we contend that it is ethical to operate to retrieve organs, under anesthesia, *prior* to treatment withdrawal. Once procuring viable vital organs under the DDR is understood as impossible to satisfy and ethically extraneous, it follows that extracting organs after withdrawing life support, as in current DCDD protocols, unnecessarily risks the viability of the organs owing to damage from warm ischemia during the time between cessation of circulation and organ extraction. In addition, procurement of hearts from patients on life support who are not "brain dead" would become more feasible by this alteration in the process of procuring vital organs. Currently, the waiting time generally precludes heart transplantation from DCDD protocols; moreover, consistent with the DDR it is difficult, if not impossible, to justify transplanting hearts when the irreversible cessation of circulation determines death. How can the heart, whose pumping is necessary for unassisted circulation, cease irreversibly in the donor but function normally in the recipient (Veatch 2008)?

Exploitation

Procuring vital organs from living patients, in violation of the DDR, has been challenged as exploiting the most vulnerable patients. The specter of exploitation was first raised by Hans Jonas in two papers written during the early stage of transplanting organs procured from "brain-dead" donors (Jonas 1970, 1974; Miller 2009b). Jonas is notable both for correctly recognizing that these individuals remained alive, in view of their continuing biological functioning while on life support, and in absolutely opposing procurement of their organs for transplantation on the basis that this involved instrumentally treating a human being as a thing, and thus using the person merely as a means to save another's life. In typically colorful language, he described organ procurement from a "brain-dead" patient as "using him as a mine" (Jonas 1970). The President's Council on Bioethics (2008), in its recent "white paper" *Controversies in the Determination of Death*, echoes this charge of exploitation in criticizing those who argue that we should dispense with the DDR. To abandon the DDR would mean that "*a living human being* may be used merely as a *means* for another human being's *ends*, losing his or her own life in the process" (President's Council 2008, 71). In his personal statement, appended to the white paper, Edmund Pellegrino, Chairman of the Council, declared that "eliminating the DDR promises a future of moral and legal chaos. Above all, it exposes the vulnerable or gullible patient to an increased danger of exploitation for the benefit of others" (President's Council 2008, 113).

We contend that the charge of exploitation is misplaced. Vital organ donation from still-living patients with prior valid decisions to withdraw LST clearly contravenes the DDR. As argued above, however, when the decision to donate vital organs is conditional on and subsequent to the decision to withdraw LST, no patient is being sacrificed to save the life of another. Procuring vital organs in the context of a prior valid decision to withdraw LST, coupled with the consent to donate, undercuts the claim that these patients are being treated merely as a means to supply organs for others in need.

In his influential analysis of the concept of exploitation, Wertheimer (1996) defines exploitation paradigmatically as one person *unfairly* taking advantage of another. It is important to note that taking advantage of another is not *ipso facto* exploitation; rather, unfairness in taking advantage constitutes exploitation.

Hence, the fact that life-saving transplantation of vital organs takes advantage of the situation of the donor who no longer needs these organs, in view of the plan to stop life support, does not, in itself, constitute exploitation. Wertheimer discusses two types of exploitation: harmful and mutually beneficial exploitation. In harmful exploitation, A takes advantage of B in a way that harms B and violates B's rights. In mutually beneficial exploitation, the unfairness concerns the distribution of benefits and burdens between the two parties. If people have an inalienable right not to be killed, then vital organ donation from living patients would be harmful exploitation. There is no reason here to delve into the philosophically controversial issue of whether any rights are inalienable. Recognizing the legitimacy of withdrawing life-sustaining treatment (understood as causing death) with valid consent suffices to demonstrate that the right not to be killed is not inalienable. Therefore, the fact that abandoning the DDR would involve killing patients does not make this practice necessarily harmful exploitation that violates their right not to be killed. Furthermore, we have argued that limiting vital organ donation to patients with prior valid decisions to withdraw LST means that they will not be harmed or wronged by procuring organs with valid consent, provided that adequate anesthesia is maintained during organ extraction and treatment withdrawal.

Vital organ donation can be a mutually beneficial transaction between donor and recipient. The patient-donors will soon die and so rarely will be able to obtain any (temporary) psychic benefit from knowing that their organs will be used to save the life of another, as they are usually mentally incapacitated at the time that the decision is made to donate. However, if patients have a strong preference that their organs be used to save others' lives, then doing so is a benefit to them. Moreover, we don't regard charitable acts, which benefit recipients even at some sacrifice to donors, as involving exploitation, so long as they were freely undertaken. There need be nothing unfair in the transaction. In vital organ donation some potential sacrifice in the goal of achieving a peaceful and dignified death may be entailed by undertaking organ extraction during the process of dying, but the patient or surrogate who consents to the donation has judged this sacrifice to be justified for the sake of saving another's life. The organ extraction is made legitimate by the consent of the donor or surrogates acting on the donor's behalf, as well as by measures to ensure comfort and respectful treatment of the patient, within the constraints of surgery to procure organs.

Slippery Slope

It might be objected that despite our arguments calling into question the rationale for the DDR, it remains necessary as a "moral compass." Without the DDR, there is no way to place acceptable limits on the scope of legitimate vital organ donation. As posed by the President's Council on Bioethics (2008, 72), "[i]f a patient need not be dead in order to be eligible for such life-ending organ donations, where would the ethical line be drawn?" Absent the DDR, what would ethically preclude killing of the mentally retarded (with parental consent), or of healthy persons with their own consent, for the sake of providing "the gift of life" to others?

A reasonable line can be drawn by limiting vital organ donation to patients with prior justified plans to withdraw life-sustaining treatment. Moreover, as indicated above, guidelines should require that the decision to withdraw life-sustaining treatment be made entirely independent of any decision about organ donation. Nevertheless, ethical worries might arise concerning pressure being put on patients or families to procure organs from those who are being maintained on life-sustaining treatment. These worries generally would be misplaced in the case of patients diagnosed as "brain dead." Although not biologically dead, such patients remain in an irreversible coma, with no prospect of recovery. Accordingly, in view of the permanent loss of consciousness, it is reasonable to hold that the person who previously occupied the still-living body has ceased to exist. Absent belief in the value of maintaining merely vegetative human life, the lack of any prospect of recovering mental life precludes the possibility that brain-dead patients can be harmed or wronged by extracting vital organs prior to stopping life-sustaining treatment. Additionally, the requirement of consent protects patients and families from lethal organ procurement that violates their religious or personal beliefs. In the situation of vital organ donation from such patients without the DDR, organs would be procured as currently practiced, though without the need for a prior declaration of death. In the case of other irreversibly compromised patients on life support, who do not meet the criteria for "brain death," the potential for illegitimate pressure to donate organs would be no different in principle than what families of patients currently face in the context of DCDD protocols, which require a prior decision to withdraw treatment. Whether life support is stopped before or after organs are retrieved from these patients, the necessary prior decision to withdraw treatment must satisfy standard ethical criteria and appropriate oversight: it reflects, or is consistent with, the preferences of the patient; the treatment is judged to be more burdensome than beneficial; or continued treatment would be futile. Any lingering doubts about the legitimacy of the prior decision to withdraw treatment, necessary to make vital organ donation permissible according to the position that we propose, might be addressed by means of ethics consultation.

A more general slippery slope concern is that legitimating vital organ donation from still-living individuals devalues human life by treating them in a way that is appropriate only for genuinely dead bodies. Insofar as this concern reflects commitment to the norm that it is always wrong to intentionally kill innocent human beings, we have addressed it in Chapters 1 and 2. Strict commitment to this norm would require abandoning the routine practice of withdrawing LST and thereby causing death—a practice that is generally thought to be ethically justified. Moreover, vital organ donation should be seen as giving due respect to the value of human life. We have argued that when made conditional on a prior decision to withdraw LST and valid consent to donate, procuring vital organs before life support is stopped does no harm or wrong to the patient-donor and permits a life-saving transplantation for the recipient. To prohibit vital organ donation, because it causes death to the donor, would devalue the lives of potential recipients who will die in the absence of transplantation. Prohibiting a harmless commission—the act of procuring vital organs from still-living patients under the justificatory conditions that we have specified—would entail a harmful omission of life-saving vital organ transplantation.

One way of protecting against a slide down the slippery slope would be to limit vital organ donation from still-living patients to exactly the same pool of donors as in the current practice of transplantation. However, the logic of our argument justifying vital organ donation without the DDR would definitely expand the eligible pool of donors to all patients on life support with valid prior decisions to stop treatment, and consent to donate, as long as their medical condition would not preclude organ viability. For example, patients in a persistent vegetative state, such as Nancy Cruzan, could become vital organ donors, following a decision to stop artificial nutrition and hydration. One difference between these patients and those on mechanical ventilation is that the former do not die a short interval after life support is withdrawn. It may take up to 2 weeks or more for these patients to die from dehydration. Yet it is difficult to see how this difference might be ethically significant. Given the decision to stop LST, no harm or wrong is done to the patient by a life-terminating procurement of vital organs rather than waiting until the patient dies from dehydration. Moreover, on the assumption that these patients are permanently unconscious, they have no interests that would be set back by ending their lives.

Although we find this argument for expanding the pool of organ donors compelling, we suggest caution in moving in this direction. Given the radical theoretical change in abandoning the DDR, it is prudent to restrict the donor pool so that it coincides with current practice until the public and clinicians become comfortable with the ethical rationale for vital organ donation from still-living donors.

Professional Integrity

Vital organ donation from still-living patients faces another pair of objections that warrants careful consideration. On the one hand, how can it be justifiable for physicians to remove vital organs from still-living donors? On the other hand, the limitation of vital organ donation to patients on life support is morally arbitrary: why shouldn't healthy persons be able to make a self-sacrificing organ donation to save the life of a loved one? To answer these queries requires revisiting the issue of the professional integrity of clinicians that we discussed in Chapter 2 relating to active euthanasia. A comprehensive ethical account of vital organ donation requires attention to professional integrity, just as it does for active euthanasia. Assessment of the interests and rights of the patient is necessary, but not sufficient, to justify these practices. Attention also must be devoted to the role morality of clinicians engaged in organ procurement and transplantation. We shall argue that the professional integrity of clinicians is compatible with vital organ donation under the ethical framework that we have developed; however, it will not permit life-ending organ donation from healthy individuals.

In discussing professional integrity with respect to vital organ donation, it helps to set the stage by discussing donation of kidneys and other body parts by healthy donors. This has become standard practice within medicine, such that the professional integrity concerns that this practice raises may be obscured from view. As a rule, clinical medicine is governed by patient-centered beneficence and nonmaleficence. This means that risks of diagnostic procedures and treatments are justified by the proportional prospect of therapeutic benefit to the patient. The practice of operating on a healthy person to remove a kidney, in order to transplant it in a recipient, falls outside this standard framework of medical risk–benefit assessment. It imposes risks of harm to a healthy person in order to benefit a patient in need of transplantation. How can it be justifiable for a physician, dedicated to the medical best interests of patients, to perform such an operation? Although psychic benefits may accrue to healthy donors, there is no way that removing a kidney can be considered in their medical best interests. To be sure, donating blood also is not in donors' medical best interests, but there is little risk of harm in this practice. Shouldn't the physician's duty to "do no harm" preclude operations to extract kidneys from healthy donors? Donation of organs and tissue from healthy individuals counts as an exception to the standard patient-centered application of the principles of beneficence and nonmaleficence within medicine. It is justified by placing strict limits on the level of harm to the donor, such that risks of mortality and serious morbidity are relatively low, and by requiring valid informed consent.

Even with careful screening, risks from kidney donation cannot be eliminated entirely. According to a recent systematic review of a large cohort of kidney donors compared with a matched sample of healthy individuals, the risk of death within 90 days following donor nephrectomy was 3.1 per 10,000 donors. The 90-day risk of death in the comparison group was 0.4 per 10,000

(Segev et al. 2010). However, longer term (12 year) follow-up indicated similar or lower mortality for kidney donors. These data do not reflect burdens, discomfort, and complications requiring medical attention following kidney donation.

Medical limitations routinely placed on eligibility for kidney donation reflect concerns for professional integrity relating to intentionally causing harm to healthy individuals. Prospective kidney donors undergo an extensive medical and psychological assessment prior to organ procurement. In this process, they are assessed for the potential for either medical or psychological harm from the procedure. With respect to avoiding medical harm, they are assessed for their risk to develop renal failure on the basis of having only one kidney. Patients with hypertension or vascular anomalies to the remaining kidney are generally considered to be at unacceptable risk. Similarly, an obese person might be considered to be at an unacceptable risk for complications from anesthesia or postoperative wound infection.

If donating kidneys from healthy individuals were governed purely by ethical considerations of autonomy and benefiting others, then these concerns about harm would not count as ethical constraints on donation. Instead, individuals would be allowed to donate as long as they understood and accepted the risks. We regard such constraints of professional integrity as ethically appropriate. Individuals are not entitled to receive from physicians whatever medical interventions they request; and physicians should decline to comply with requests that would violate their professional integrity, owing to valid concerns regarding inflicting disproportionate harm.

Is vital organ donation from still-living patients compatible with professional integrity? If we set aside for the moment the fact that vital organ donation from living patients involves interventions that cause the patient's death (or are incompatible with their continued survival), this practice is easier to justify with respect to professional integrity than donations of kidneys from healthy individuals. In accordance with our recommended ethical framework of making vital organ donation conditional on a prior planned withdrawal of LST, there is no harm to the donor from procuring organs prior to stopping treatment. However, clearly, it is the connection with causing death that poses concerns for professional integrity. Yet since it is ethical for physicians to withdraw LST with death as the outcome—indeed, it is obligatory to respect valid refusals of treatment—there is no necessary ethical bar to procuring vital organs before stopping such treatment when the patient or surrogate has given valid consent for donation. Moreover, we argued in Chapter 2 that active euthanasia as a last resort is compatible with professional integrity. Accordingly, it is difficult to see how the role morality of medicine, understood from a critical perspective that rejects the traditional norm that doctors must never intentionally cause the death of their patients, would preclude vital organ donation from still-living patients, when it is conditional on valid decisions to withdraw LST.

To be sure, both withdrawing LST and active euthanasia are directed at benefiting the patient by relieving suffering (associated with continued life support and the patient's incurable condition) and/or by terminating a life that with respect to the well-being of the patient is no longer considered worth living. Vital organ donation is not patient centered in this respect, though it may respect the preferences of the patient. But because it poses no harm to the donor in the context of a prior plan to withdraw LST, and it provides life-saving or enhancing therapeutic benefit for the recipient, vital organ donation from still-living patients is compatible with professional integrity. By virtue of not harming the donor, this practice does not contravene the goals of medicine; and it promotes the goals of medicine by being instrumental to the therapeutic benefit for the recipient.

Because procuring vital organs is not an intervention in the service of patient care with respect to the donor, it might be seen as contrary to the duties incumbent on physicians in pursuing medical goals. Particularly relevant in this respect are the duties of avoiding disproportionate harm to patients that are not balanced by the prospect of compensating medical benefits and fidelity to the therapeutic relationship with patients in need of care. The donor is not harmed by vital organ donation in the context of a planned withdrawal of LST. Although procuring organs for transplantation can by no means be seen as therapeutic for the donor, the lack of harm from the donation, coupled with adequate anesthesia to block any suffering from the process, makes this practice not inconsistent with fidelity to patients. Although outside the context of standard medical care, procuring vital organs from still-living patient-donors on life support is compatible with professional integrity. Once understood that it is ethically acceptable for physicians to cause the death of patients in a range of end-of-life situations, physician involvement in vital organ donation with still-living patients, subject to necessary ethical constraints, is no less justifiable than other medical practices that involve the donation of organs and tissues for the benefit of others.

Another way of posing and rebutting the challenge to professional integrity is the following. It might be thought that the medical interests of still-living patients on life support with the potential to supply vital organs compete with the medical interests of potential transplant recipients. The former would be killed in the process of organ procurement; the latter would be given life-saving transplantation. Because it would be unethical for physicians to sacrifice the interests of one patient to serve the interests of another, vital organ donation from still-living patients violates professional integrity. We have argued, however, that patient-donors on life support with a prior plan to withdraw treatment and valid consent to donate organs have no interests that are set back by organ procurement in view of this prior decision. Hence, physicians do not face competing interests under this scenario and, therefore, would not be involved in sacrificing the interests of one patient to serve those of another. In sum, professional integrity is not compromised.

In contrast, participation in a self-sacrificing vital organ donation by a healthy individual interested in saving the life of a loved one or performing an altruistic act would be very difficult, if not impossible, to square with the professional integrity of clinicians. Yet this situation poses a clash of ethical considerations. On the one hand, it is plausible to suppose that some parents, for example, might be prepared to sacrifice their lives to save the life of one of their children; and vital organ donation is one context in which this might seem an appropriate, and perhaps commendable, act. On the other hand, it seems obvious that no clinician should be obliged to comply with such a request for help in achieving vital organ transplantation. However, we are not merely arguing for the weak claim that *requiring* clinicians to perform vital organ procurement from a healthy person would violate professional integrity. Rather, the issue we are facing here is whether it can be *permissible* for a clinician to comply with the request of a healthy person to undertake a lethal organ procurement. Killing a healthy person undoubtedly conflicts with the goals of medicine. This is not obviated by the requesting donor's consent. The grave, life-ending, harm to a healthy individual could not be compensated by the life-saving benefit to another in need of transplantation, especially if it may become possible for the needed organs to be obtained from a donor on life support with a plan to die by stopping treatment. Although no wrong would be done to the healthy donor, in view of valid consent, it arguably would be wrong for clinicians to perform a life-ending operation on a healthy person.

Irrespective of consent, professional integrity-preserving constraints on physicians procuring vital organs from still-living patients parallel constraints on physicians performing active euthanasia. Some might, nonetheless, argue that it is permissible for clinicians to participate in vital organ donation from healthy donors, given scrupulous informed consent, out of respect for their autonomy, on the ground that this consideration should outweigh any ethical qualms relating to professional integrity. We disagree that autonomy, in this situation, has an overriding moral force that trumps considerations of professional integrity. In any case, we suspect that few, if any, clinicians would be willing to take part in an operation to procure vital organs from a healthy person.

A full consideration of tensions between autonomy and professional integrity is outside the scope of our inquiry. It is worth noting, however, that it is reasonable to place limits on the justificatory power of consent. Consent generally creates *moral transformation*: it makes conduct permissible that otherwise would be prohibited (Kleinig 2010). For example, consent marks the difference between slavery and employment, theft and borrowing, rape and consensual sexual intercourse, and treating patients as human guinea pigs and ethical clinical research. It might be thought, accordingly, that as long as valid consent to donate vital organs has been provided by a patient (or surrogate), physicians are thereby permitted to procure these organs, even though death will ensue as a result. Likewise, consent should be sufficient to justify active euthanasia. The reigning theory of consent, which views consent as an *autonomous authorization* (Faden and Beauchamp 1986), arguably reinforces this conception of the justificatory force of consent. Consent, however, is a bilateral transaction (Miller and Wertheimer 2010). We need to consider ethical constraints on the one who receives consent as well as the autonomy of the consenter. When A gives valid consent for B to do X, it means that no wrong is done to A if B does X. It does not follow that B, in all cases, is permitted to do X. Specifically, professional integrity places constraints on what physicians are permitted to do, independent of the consent of patients. Outside the realm of medicine, it is also reasonable for the law and morality to place limits on what consent can justify with respect to behavior that results in grave harm (Bergelson 2010).

These considerations of professional integrity further help to address the slippery slope concerns that we discussed in the previous section. The role morality of medicine places strict constraints on vital organ donation from still-living patients. The argument against assisting in a self-sacrificing organ donation from a healthy person would also apply to procuring vital organs from a mentally retarded individual, and the prohibition would be strengthened in this case by the absence of valid consent on the part of the donor.

How should we think about the case of a terminally ill patient who wishes to die and to donate vital organs (assuming that they would be viable)? If active euthanasia would be ethically appropriate in this case, which according to the argument of Chapter 2 would require unbearable suffering that could not be otherwise adequately relieved, what would be the ethical objection to procuring vital organs as the means of ending the patient's life? In this case, the decision to donate would not be conditional on a prior plan to withdraw LST but would be conditional on a prior plan to die by active euthanasia. Suppose further that the request to donate was made by a patient living in a country, such as the Netherlands and Belgium, that legally permits euthanasia by lethal injection. In this particular context, the logic of our ethical framework for vital organ donation would permit organ procurement in this case, and no valid considerations of professional integrity would preclude it. Thus, we conclude that in this narrowly circumscribed situation, vital organ donation would be ethically acceptable. In fact, vital organ donation and active euthanasia have been combined in Belgium. Curiously from the perspective of our ethical framework, organs were procured after the patient who received a lethal injection was declared dead in accordance with circulatory criteria under a DCDD protocol (Ysebaert et al. 2009). Given the plan to cause death by lethal injection, we see no ethical purpose in attempting to comply with the DDR, especially as this risks the optimal viability of the organs to be transplanted.

Another challenging issue relating to professional integrity and vital organ donation posed by our ethical framework is the legitimacy of procuring organs in connection with capital punishment. Considerable critical attention has been evoked by the practice of organ donation in connection with execution of prisoners in China (Diflo 2004; Wang and Wang 2010). Here we focus on a thought experiment aimed at analyzing and assessing the force of professional integrity in the context of physician participation in capital punishment. Suppose that a death-row prisoner, slated to be killed by lethal injection, decides that he wants to donate his organs. Recognizing the magnitude of his guilt for murder, he wishes to make some good come out of the ending of his life. Would it be ethical for transplant clinicians to procure organs from this prisoner? We assume that the organ procurement, undertaken in connection with the sentence of death, would take place in the operating room of a hospital.

If organ procurement was considered ethical in this situation, consistent with our ethical framework, the ideal way to do so would be to anesthetize the prisoner and extract the organs while he remains alive. Given the conviction for a capital crime and the judicially imposed sentence of death, the prisoner will die regardless of whether organs are procured. In this scenario, and in view of the prisoner's informed consent to donate, no harm or wrong is done to the prisoner by procuring organs prior to death. The question we pose is whether the organ procurement is compatible with the professional integrity of transplant clinicians.

In addressing this question, it is essential to bracket the ethics of capital punishment. If capital punishment is wrong, then it is at least prima facie wrong for doctors to participate, in any way, in capital punishment. But if capital punishment is not wrong, can it be ethical for clinicians to participate via procuring organs? In the case as we have described it, the organ procurement cannot be isolated from the execution, as it is the extracting of organs that causes death. Professional codes of ethics for physicians have uniformly prohibited participation in capital punishment (Dworkin 2002). Although this suggests that there may be good ethical reasons for considering participation in capital punishment as contrary to the role morality of medicine, the code prohibition by itself is not decisive. Codes of medical ethics generally prohibit active euthanasia by lethal injection, but we have argued that this practice is not inherently contrary to professional integrity. We need to examine the goals of medicine and the role-specific duties incumbent on physicians in practicing medicine to determine whether they would permit organ procurement from a prisoner condemned to death.

The prisoner is not a patient of the transplant clinicians and organ procurement is not in the medical interests of the prisoner. This, however, is also true of "brain-dead" donors and those who donate under DCDD protocols, as well as healthy donors. We argued above that the goals of medicine are not violated with respect to procurement of vital organs from still-living donors conditional on a prior valid decision to withdraw LST. But there is a difference of potential ethical significance between the capital punishment case and vital organ donation for patients on life support. Although in our ethical framework, the life-terminating procurement of organs for these latter donors is not done for their medical benefit, the withdrawal of treatment, on which vital organ procurement is conditional, is medically appropriate. It avoids harm to the patient from continued, nonbeneficial and burdensome life support, and it respects the patient's preferences or values. In other words, the decision to stop treatment, which opens up the ethical possibility of organ procurement prior to death, is a patient-centered decision. In contrast, the decision to execute the prisoner, which is the precondition for organ procurement in the case under consideration, is not in any sense for the benefit of the prisoner. This suggests that the duty of fidelity to the therapeutic relationship with the patient might be considered as having differential implications for vital organ donation from patients on life support as compared with the capital punishment case. To repeat, in neither situation is the death-causing organ procurement a therapeutic act for the donor. However, the prior plan to withdraw LST certainly falls within the scope of fidelity to the therapeutic relationship with the patient. When continued treatment is no longer therapeutic for the patient, and the patient or surrogate has decided to stop treatment, then fidelity to the patient calls for withdrawing life support. Patient-centered fidelity does not get a foothold in the capital punishment case. On the other hand, patient-centered fidelity has no bearing either on kidney donations from healthy individuals. These individuals are patients only in the sense that they are undergoing an operation, but one that is not for their benefit. The same is true of the prisoner-donor. In both cases, the organ donation reflects the donors' decision to help another. Shouldn't this decision of the prisoner, who believes that his life, as a whole, will have gone better by virtue of donating his organs, deserve respect?

Stronger concern relating to professional integrity is evoked by recognition that by intervening to cause the death of the prisoner, pursuant to the judicial sentence of death, the transplant clinicians, in effect, become agents of the state in performing capital punishment. In other words, they are the executioners. It seems essentially foreign to the ethos of medicine for doctors to become executioners (Miller and Brody 1995; Dworkin 2002). If physician participation in capital punishment is contrary to professional ethics, it would seem that the same should apply when the prisoner's judicially mandated death is caused by organ procurement.

Might this concern be allayed by arranging the organ donation consistent with the way in which procurement has proceeded in Belgium in conjunction with active euthanasia (as described above)? Execution by lethal injection would be performed prior to organ procurement, which would be governed by a DCDD protocol. In that situation, extracting organs arguably would be subsequent to execution, and therefore the transplant clinicians, strictly speaking, would not be participating in capital punishment. The problem with this proposal is that it is predicated on the claim that the prisoner-donor is dead, consistent with the DDR, at the time that the organs are procured. Because we have argued that we cannot be certain that cessation of circulation is irreversible in the case of standard DCDD protocols, it is not clear that the organ procurement can be isolated from the execution. On balance, in light of our ethical framework, we do not recommend permitting organ procurement from prisoners condemned to death. Yet we recognize that reasonable persons might well differ on this issue, as this practice can provide life-saving transplantation without harm or wrong to the prisoner and respects his autonomous choice. Greater ethical attention to this complex issue is warranted, including the question of whether professional integrity has sufficient moral force to preclude absolutely organ procurement connected with capital punishment.

Is It Necessary to Limit Vital Organ Donation to Patients on Life Support?

At the end of this lengthy consideration of objections to our ethical framework for justifying vital organ donation without the DDR, the question remains why it should be limited only to patients with a prior decision to withdraw LST. Consider the case of a 61-year-old man with amyotrophic lateral sclerosis (diagnosed 2 years previously) living in the state of Georgia who expressed a wish to end his life by donating his organs (CNN Wire Staff 2010). He is not ventilator dependent. If he were on a ventilator and had made a competent choice to stop LST, then he would qualify for vital organ donation immediately prior to treatment withdrawal according to our ethical framework. Isn't it ethically arbitrary to make the legitimacy of vital organ donation from a still-living individual depend on whether he is on life support? Although less problematic than a self-sacrificing organ donation from a healthy person, this case poses concerns of professional integrity in that organ procurement would involve clinicians in ending the life of an individual who might continue to live for a number of years. The patient's prognosis is ethically relevant to complying with a request to die by means of organ donation, analogous to comparable concerns relating to active euthanasia. As argued above, in the case of a patient on life support who validly refuses continuing treatment, death will ensue from the treatment withdrawal, obviating concerns of professional integrity for procuring vital organs prior to stopping the ventilator.

We don't claim that there are clear ethical principles that *dictate* this constraint on vital organ donation. Indeed, we have discussed above a case of vital organ procurement from a terminally ill patient not on life support that seems ethically appropriate in the context of a plan for active euthanasia. Although making vital organ donation conditional on a prior valid decision to withdraw LST means that procuring vital organs before stopping treatment will not harm the patient, there may be other situations in which a patient chooses to donate vital organs that also could reasonably be described as not causing harm. Nevertheless, we submit that a variety of practical and policy considerations support this constraint on vital organ donation (at least in the context of jurisdictions that have not legalized active euthanasia). First, the situations in which procuring vital organs from still-living patients would be justified under our ethical framework coincide with the situations that are now justified with respect to the DDR: patients with a diagnosis of "brain death" and those on life support who qualify for DCDD protocols. (We noted above a possible exception for patients with a diagnosis of persistent vegetative state with valid prior decisions to stop artificial nutrition and hydration, who would not qualify for current DCDD protocols.) In essence, we are offering an alternative ethical justification of our current practices because the established ethical rationale in terms of the DDR is based on false judgments that the donors are dead or known to be dead. Though radical with respect to the underlying ethical premises justifying vital organ donation, our ethical framework is relatively conservative in practice. It merely dispenses with prior declarations of death, which represent fictions and fudging of the truth on our account, and licenses procuring vital organs prior to stopping life support. Second, the constraint on vital organ donation that makes it conditional on a valid prior decision to withdraw LST bars problematic and clearly unethical organ procurement from incompetent individuals who are not on life support. As such, it guards against a slippery slope to exploitation of the vulnerable. Third, it preserves the professional integrity of clinicians, as we argued above. Finally, related to this last point, it recognizes limits on autonomy in justifying harmful, death-causing interventions: for example, consent is not sufficient to justify physicians performing life-ending organ procurement in the case of healthy persons.

ABANDONING THE DISTINCTION BETWEEN LIVE AND CADAVERIC DONATION

The prevailing ethical thinking regarding organ donation has relied on a sharp distinction between live and "cadaveric" organ donation. Vital organ donations have been held justifiable only in the case of dead donors. This distinction is challenged, however, by recognition that current practices in fact violate the DDR. Moreover, our justification of vital organ donation without the DDR brings the ethical rationale for this practice in line with the standard rationale for current practices of live donation of organs and tissues, such as kidneys and bone marrow. In the latter case, organ donation from a healthy person is justified by the absence of undue harm and valid consent. It obviously is not possible to avoid any harm to the donor in the context of an operation to extract a kidney. But the potential for mortality and serious morbidity is judged to be sufficiently low to warrant an operation that can enhance and help prolong the life of the recipient. In the case of vital organ donation, we have argued that harm to the donor can be avoided when the procurement of organs is conditional on a planned withdrawal of LST and adequate anesthesia is administered. There remains some potential burden on the patient's family from combining the end-of-life care with organ procurement. This burden, however, is justified and outweighed by the psychic benefits deriving from the decision to donate, the prior preferences and values of the donor (when applicable), and the great benefit to another that can come from transplantation. As in the case of current practices of live kidney donation, live vital organ donation would require valid consent.

The implication of our ethical framework with respect to organ donation in general is that whether the donor is alive or dead has no ethical salience for the justification of procuring organs. Rather, we look to circumstances under which donors will not be harmed, or not unduly harmed, by organ donation. In the case of vital organ donation, this turns out to be situations in which ending the patient's life in the process of procuring vital organs will not set back any interests of the donor. Either they have no interests that can be set back by death, owing to the irreversible loss of consciousness, or they are on a planned, imminent trajectory toward death, owing to a prior valid decision to stop LST. In fact, these two situations are closely connected. Those donors who have irreversibly lost the capacity for consciousness are also being sustained by life support. In both cases, an independent plan to withdraw treatment precedes organ procurement. The distinction between live and cadaveric donation is not completely abandoned, however, as tissues, such as corneas, can be procured from dead bodies.

NOTHING IS LOST

It is instructive to examine the logic of an argument analogous to our justification of vital organ donation without the DDR, as it helps bring into focus some additional relevant issues and points of clarification. In a subtle and carefully crafted defense of embryonic stem cell research using spare embryos produced in the context of in vitro fertilization, Gene Outka appeals to the principle that "nothing is lost." Outka (2002) builds on the work of Paul Ramsey, who argued in favor of an exception to the absolute prohibition of intentional killing of innocent human beings under two conditions: "(1) the innocent will die in any case; and (2) other innocent life will be saved" (193). Outka explicates the nothing is lost (NIL) principle as one in which "unless one directly kills one of the parties, one cannot save the life of another. This allows the claim that one *would* save both if one *could*" (195). The spare embryos are destined to be destroyed—"They will be *lost* no matter what one does" (204). Accordingly, it is permissible for investigators to use them in embryonic stem cell research aimed at curing life-threatening diseases—use that will result in their destruction.

Another example of the NIL principle is the following. During the Nazi era, a group of Jews is hiding at a farm house. They receive word that the Gestapo is on the way to investigate whether Jews are being harbored in the area. They hide in a cellar that is accessed by a hidden trap door. Among the group is a baby who begins to cry and can't be consoled. Hearing the voices of the Gestapo officers, the baby's mother smothers the child who dies as a result. On the reasonable assumption that all would die if discovered by the Gestapo, the baby would die in any case and the lives of the others could be saved as a result of smothering the baby. Assuming further that there were no other available means of keeping the baby quiet, many would see this tragic killing as justified (Greene 2009).

Though the fact patterns of these two instances of the NIL principle are very different from each other and from vital organ donation, the analogies between the justifications of these cases and our account of vital organ donation from still-living patients are obvious. In the context of a legitimate plan to withdraw LST, the (innocent) patient will die soon regardless of whether organs are procured before stopping treatment. Just as nothing is lost in destroying embryos within valuable stem cell research, provided that the embryos are spare ones that are slated to be destroyed, so nothing is lost in procuring vital organs from patients on life support in the context of prior plans to withdraw LST. Nothing is lost in vital organ donation from still-living patients on life support because they have no interests that are set back in organ procurement prior to a planned treatment withdrawal.

Interestingly, in passing, Outka explicitly rejects extending the NIL principle to procuring organs from living patients who are terminally ill or permanently comatose (205). However, he does not engage the issue of whether current donors of vital organs are, in fact, dead. There would be no need to invoke the NIL principle if current practices were consistent with the DDR. But if there is no way to achieve the life-saving transplantation of vital organs from the (truly) dead, then it is not clear why the NIL principle should bar vital organ donation under the justificatory conditions that we have set out. In rejecting this application of the NIL principle, Outka merely asserts that "It is *impermissible* to destroy *any* entity for body parts who has an agential history even if he or she does not now have any considerable future" (205). Given the decision by the patient or surrogate on behalf of the patient to withdraw LST, these patients, and potential donors, will die in any case, and the use of their organs can save the lives of others, thus satisfying the two conditions for the NIL principle. Furthermore, clinicians would save the lives both of the potential donors and the potential recipients if they could. But the former have dire medical conditions that preclude restoration to any satisfactory quality of life, and valid decisions have been made to stop their LST, leading to death. The latter's lives can be saved only if they receive vital organs, which, as a matter of fact, can be procured only from still-living patients. Accordingly, it is not clear why the NIL principle applies to embryonic stem cell research but not to vital organ donation. (Outka does not discuss a case such as the smothered baby, though it satisfies the two conditions for the NIL principle specified by Ramsey.)

The first condition of the NIL principle—that the innocent will die in any case—needs to be specified carefully. Obviously, the fact that all of us will eventually die does not license forcefully extracting organs from one healthy person to save the lives of several others. The idea that nothing will be lost helps in suggesting the necessary specification of this principle for the situation of vital organ donation. It is impossible to hold that nothing is lost when a healthy person, even with a requirement for stringent and carefully vetted consent, chooses to sacrifice his or her life by means of vital organ donation to save the life of another. This person would not die in any case, but only as a result of implementing the decision to donate his or her vital organs to save the life of another. The point is not that a life worth living is ended, for this is true of the smothered baby; rather, it is the fact that under the situation in question death of the innocent is bound to occur, independent of the death-causing intervention that falls under the NIL principle. In our ethical justification of vital organ donation without the DDR, the prior decision to withdraw LST makes death imminent and unavoidable. Accordingly, no harm comes to the patient, and the patient loses nothing, from lethal organ procurement prior to LST, provided that adequate anesthesia is administered.

The NIL principle, by definition, links the lack of loss to the innocent who is killed, under a given set of circumstances, to the life-saving gain to another made possible by virtue of the former's death. Nothing is lost coincides with something vital being gained. This entails an important corollary to the NIL principle, which Outka does not explicitly consider: under situations in which the NIL principle applies, *something is lost* if life-ending interventions are *not* performed. Valuable embryonic stem cell research will not be performed unless embryos are destroyed in the process, nor will vital organs be procured and transplanted unless still-living patients are donors. Failure to conduct the research and perform the transplantations entails significant losses to human health and well-being.

In invoking the something is lost corollary, we imagine being admonished by the shade of Hans Jonas. At the end of a justly famous essay published in 1970 on the ethics of human experimentation, which also discussed the new neuro-logical criteria for determining death and organ transplantation, Jonas implored, "Let us not forget that progress is an optional goal, not an unconditional commitment. . . . Let us also remember that a slower progress in the conquest of disease would not threaten society, grievous as it is to those who have to deplore that their particular disease be not yet conquered, but that society would indeed be threatened by the erosion of those moral values whose loss, possibly caused by too ruthless a pursuit of scientific progress, would make its dazzling triumphs not worth having" (Jonas 1970). Reflecting on organ trans-plantation when it was still an experimental procedure, Jonas believed that pro-curing organs from patients in an irreversible coma—who were defined as dead but, in his opinion, were still-living patients—was just the sort of grave moral wrong that would make the "dazzling triumphs" of scientific progress "not worth having." Though he was mistaken in his moral assessment of vital organ donation from "brain-dead" donors (Miller 2009b), as our argument in favor of this practice implies, Jonas undoubtedly was right that progress is not morally imperative *if* it comes at the expense of violating human rights. Scientific and technological interventions aimed at promoting human well-being must be subject to deontological constraints. Care must be taken to impose appropri-ate constraints on live-saving interventions, lest wrongful killing and exploita-tion would be permitted. Our ethical framework specifies the necessary constraints.

Because the end doesn't (necessarily) justify the means, the something is lost corollary must be hedged. Indeed, it is hedged (at least in part) by the joint application of the two components of the NIL principle. It bears repeating that if nothing is lost by procuring vital organs from still-living patients on life support, in the context of valid decisions to stop treatment, then something of great importance is lost when, without compelling reasons, we refrain from procuring the organs because the patient is not dead.

The NIL principle, when applied to vital organ donation, suggests two interesting implications for our ethical framework. First, our argument in defense of vital organ donation without the DDR relies on the premise that stopping LST causes death, contrary to the standard view in medical ethics. However, it is not necessary to see withdrawing LST as causing death for the NIL principle to get a foothold. It is sufficient that the innocent patient is going to die following treatment withdrawal. This *can* be understood as merely allowing the patient to die from the underlying medical condition and still pose the nothing is lost scenario. Nothing would be lost by killing the patient in the context of procuring vital organs, as the patient will die in any case following withdrawal of life support. Nonetheless, we stand by the assertion that withdrawing LST causes death, both because we regard it as true and we believe that appealing to this true account of the consequences of withdrawing LST strengthens the argument in favor of vital organ donation despite contravening the DDR. The justifiability of causing death by stopping life support calls into question the judgment that it is necessarily wrong to cause death by procuring vital organs in the context of a prior plan of stopping treatment. This account of withdrawing LST also challenges Outka's assertion that "It is *impermissible* to destroy *any* entity for body parts who has an agential history even if he or she does not now have any considerable future." Given the justifiability of causing death by stopping LST, a cogent account needs to be supplied for why it is deemed wrong to procure vital organs before treatment is withdrawn, given the lack of harm to the patient and the application of the NIL principle.

Second, it might be thought that endorsing vital organ donation without the DDR is tantamount to endorsing active euthanasia. This is not the case. Both involve direct killing, but it does not follow that the justification of the former presupposes the justification of the latter. In accordance with the NIL principle, saving the life of another does crucial justificatory work in permitting the killing of an innocent person who will die regardless. Active euthanasia is directed at benefiting the patient, not at helping another. It therefore does not satisfy the two conditions of the NIL principle. Specifically, the NIL principle would not justify active euthanasia for patients with a valid prior decision to withdraw life support, such as a patient in a persistent vegetative state whose surrogate decides to stop artificial nutrition and hydration. One can consistently justify vital organ donation from still-living patients while rejecting entirely active euthanasia. The NIL principle helps in exhibiting this point.

Despite its close analogies with our ethical framework, we do not embrace the NIL perspective to justify vital organ donation for two reasons. First, the NIL principle, as explicated by Outka, has no reference to consent in justifying killing the innocent. We view consent as an important, if not necessary, justificatory condition for vital organ donation. Nonetheless, it is possible to add consent as a necessary condition for applying the NIL principle in some contexts. In the next section, we discuss the necessity of consent in the context of two arguments in favor of an obligation to procure vital organs.

Second, Outka's argument, invoking the NIL principle, treats justified destruction of the embryo in stem cell research as a necessary evil. His use of the NIL approach is explicitly premised on a state of moral disquiet, which he describes as "permanent unease." In other words, there is something wrong about destroying embryos, though justified when they are spare embryos from in vitro fertilization (IVF), which are otherwise slated to be destroyed. Although many would see no reason for permanent unease in destroying embryos, clearly this sense of moral disquiet is appropriate for the case of the baby killed to save the lives of a threatened group. We do not, however, view vital organ donation without the DDR in this light. We have argued that no harm or wrong is done to the patient-donor in the context of a valid prior decision to withdraw LST and appropriate consent to donate. In other words, we see no reason to regret procuring vital organs under these circumstances.

Of course, it is unfortunate that patients are in a situation in which stopping LST is judged to be desirable to protect them from harm and respect their preferences and values. This unfortunate circumstance makes it ethically possible to use their organs to save the lives of others. It doesn't follow that there is any wrong, even *pro tanto* wrong, to them in procuring their organs under the justificatory conditions that we have specified. Nor do we see any wrong involved apart from a (possible) wrong to the patient-donor. Certainly, we recognize that the vulnerable patient on LST is a human being entitled to respect and protection from harm, placing important constraints on the circumstances under which vital organs can be procured. Insofar as there is any moral disquiet hovering over vital organ donation, it relates to the *potential* for exploitation—a potential that also pertains to the current practice of DCDD protocols, nominally subject to the DDR. Outka holds that stem cell research using spare embryos is "morally tolerable, and no more" (206). We see vital organ donation from still-living patients as less ethically fraught, though highly controversial, because it conflicts with established medical ethics. In the next section, we briefly discuss more robust justificatory accounts under which vital organ procurement is regarded as obligatory and consent as thereby unnecessary.

IS THERE AN OBLIGATION TO SUPPLY VITAL ORGANS?

We have been discussing transplantation of vital organs in terms of the standard concept of *donation*. The donation model suggests that organ donation is a charitable act: there is neither a strict obligation to donate organs nor a correlative right of a needy patient to receive them. It is a gift, not something that it is owed to another who can claim it as a matter of right. Yet certainly in family contexts, people may feel obligated to donate bone marrow or a kidney to a close family member in need, just as we feel obligated to give gifts in certain social situations. Likewise, some religious and moral perspectives prescribe an obligation to make charitable donations. In none of these donation cases, however, do we see the recipient of the gift as having a right to receive it. In traditional moral terminology, if there is an obligation to make donations, it is an imperfect duty, over which the agent has discretion, not a perfect duty, such as a promise, that corresponds to a claim-right on the part of the recipient. Closely tied to the donation model is the requirement of consent. Because making available organs for transplantation to another in need is understood as a gift, over which the donor has discretion, consent is an ethically necessary condition.

The donation model has been challenged by some ethicists who argue that making organs available, at least in some circumstances, should be seen as a strict obligation owed to others in need. Two approaches have been advanced to reach this conclusion: one based on beneficence and the other on distributive justice. Nelson (2009) has suggested that supplying vital organs is analogous to providing emergency aid to people in need. We generally recognize a duty to provide aid to people in dire need during emergency situations when we have the capability to rescue them and can do so without risking substantial harm to ourselves. Transplantation of vital organs arguably falls into this moral category of a duty to rescue, notwithstanding the fact that these organs are being procured from still-living individuals, rather than from cadavers. No harm will be done to the sources of these organs, either in the case of those who are diagnosed as "brain dead" or in the context of DCDD protocols. Hence, Nelson argues that the moral default should be set in favor of organ procurement, such that affirmative consent is not required. Instead, opt-out consent may be appropriate. The logic of the argument, however, based on the appeal to a duty of rescue, might be extended to call into question any requirement of consent as a condition for vital organ procurement, especially in view of the fact that the "brain dead" and those patients on life support with a plan to withdraw treatment have no need for their organs.

Fabre (2006) argues for "confiscating cadaveric organs" on the basis of distributive justice. She sums up her argument as follows: "if the interest of the needy in leading a minimally flourishing life is important enough to be protected by a right to material resources, by way of taxation in general and financial restrictions on inheritance in particular, then the sick have a right to the organs of the dead if they need them in order to lead such a life. To put it differently, the living cannot, and do not, have any right to dispose of their body as they wish posthumously; nor do their relatives have that right" (96). Fabre assumes the standard conception of transplantation using cadaveric organs. When the sources of these organs are understood, correctly, as still living, it might be thought that the argument collapses. For instead of taking organs from dead bodies to save the lives of others in need, organs would be taken from living, vulnerable patients. Setting aside any concerns about killing, the opposing claim of bodily integrity, however, might be seen as relatively weak, insofar as the patients who would supply vital organs—the "brain dead" and those on life support for whom decisions have been made to stop treatment— have no need to retain their transplantable organs and would not be harmed by organ procurement.

Moreover, Fabre makes essentially the same argument in favor of an enforce- able claim, under distributive justice, for "confiscating live body parts" from healthy individuals, including blood, bone marrow, and even kidneys, when there is little risk of serious harm to the source of the organs. She contends that "in arguing for the compulsory taking of live body parts, I am arguing that it is unjust to deny one's organs to those who need them, even if one does not con- sent to be considered as a supplier, where what is at stake is the possibility for them to lead a minimally flourishing life, and a fortiori to survive. To put it differently: the sick, or so I argue, have a moral right against the able-bodied that the latter give them (some of) their body parts whilst alive" (100). If her arguments are sound in favor of an enforceable obligation to make available organs from what are considered cadaveric sources and from healthy persons, then these arguments could also be extended to support a policy of extracting vital organs from still-living patients on life support with plans to withdraw treatment.

The arguments of Nelson and Fabre deserve careful, critical attention, but we will not pursue them further here. Whatever theoretical merits they have need to be balanced by practical difficulties in implementing an enforceable obliga- tion to supply organs, which would disturb or outrage those opposed to organ procurement under any circumstances from still-living patients. Specifically, a policy of vital organ confiscation might influence surrogates opposed to organ procurement to insist on maintaining LST for incapacitated patients with no chance of recovery. These difficulties might be addressed by a conscientious exemption for those who have religious reasons for opposing vital organ transplantation (comparable to a conscientious exemption for required military service), but many might resist mandatory organ procurement without any provision for consent. Additionally, such a mandatory policy would require that the last moments of patients removed from life support who would be eligible for organ procurement would occur in the surgical setting of the operating room.

Advocating vital organ donation without the DDR is a sufficiently controversial prospect, without compounding the controversy by arguing for an obligation to supply organs and the abandonment of a consent requirement. We suggest, nonetheless, that these arguments in favor of an obligation to supply needed vital organs bolster the position that we are advancing here. If there are sound theoretical reasons, grounded in beneficence and distributive justice, for the strong position that there is an obligation to supply vital organs, without being conditioned on consent, then this makes all the more powerful the argument for the weaker position that vital organ donation is *permissible* from still-living patients on life support, for whom valid decisions to withdraw treatment have been made, when backed by consent to donate. Although it would be reasonable to claim that other things being equal, viable vital organs ought to be donated when patients no longer have any need for them, we believe that, on balance, an enforceable obligation to supply vital organs imposes too great an infringement on the autonomy of patients and their families.

Assuming that consent is required for vital organ donation, considerable attention will need to be devoted to how it is legitimate to obtain it. As we have indicated above, current practices of obtaining consent, both as an advance directive and contemporaneously, will need to be transformed to reflect the fact that donors are not dead immediately prior to the time when vital organs are extracted. Furthermore, various arguments that support making the default in favor of donation, with an opportunity to opt out, as well as those that attempt to justify conscripting organs, without any need for consent, will no longer have persuasive force insofar as they rely on donors being dead. For example, one recent article argues for organ conscription based on an analogy with mandatory autopsies (Hershenov and Delaney 2009). Autopsies are necessarily predicated on the body being dead; hence, this argument becomes irrelevant.

We will not pursue any further here the process of informed consent for vital organ donation, as our focus is on laying the foundation for an alternative ethical framework justifying vital organ donation without the DDR. The project of reshaping informed consent becomes otiose if either our claims about the still-living status of current vital organ donors are not sound or no satisfactory alternative ethical framework can be developed, leading to the conclusion that vital organ donation is unethical. Accordingly, we see the issue of redefining informed consent as a project for the future, when widespread support exists for reconstructing the ethics of vital organ donation.

AS GOOD AS DEAD

We began this chapter by posing the conundrum of procuring organs from "brain-dead" individuals, as formulated by Greenberg in an article entitled "As Good as Dead." The phrase "as good as dead" has also appeared a few times in the text. This might be seen as no more than a catchy label, not to be taken seriously, or as objectionable by virtue of implying that some living human beings ought to be treated as if they were dead. We suggest, however, that when applied to the situation of vital organ donation, "as good as dead" can be explicated in a meaningful way that both reflects the reality of our current practices and encapsulates the argument of this chapter.

To be as good as dead obviously is not the same as being dead; otherwise the phrase would be useless. An individual is as good as dead when he is in a situation in which it is appropriate, in some respect, to treat him as if he were dead. This does not mean that it is appropriate to treat him in all respects in the same way as we treat a dead human body. Corpses are ready to be buried or cremated, which is not true of individuals who are as good as dead. For example, some might see individuals in a permanent vegetative state as being as good as dead, such that it would be legitimate to end their lives by stopping life-sustaining treatment or by active euthanasia and also to procure vital organs from them. It does not follow that it would be appropriate to bury or cremate them while they are breathing spontaneously. In other words, it makes sense to say that some individuals are as good as dead in some respects but not in others. Our concern in this chapter is organ donation. When you are dead you can't be harmed by extracting your organs to save (or enhance) the lives of others. Nor can you be wronged if valid consent has been obtained for organ donation. We have argued that there are conditions under which living individuals can donate vital organs while satisfying the ethical constraints of not being harmed or wronged. These individuals are as good as dead.

There are two different ways to be as good as dead with respect to procuring vital organs. Individuals diagnosed as "brain dead" may be seen as good as dead by virtue of their *status*. These individuals are known (with practical certainty) to be permanently unconscious. They are alive but have no experience and no chance of recovering it. This makes their situation subjectively indistinguishable from death. Describing the dread of death in his poem "Aubade," Philip Larkin, wrote, "That this is what we fear—no sight, no sound,/No touch or taste or smell, nothing to think with,/Nothing to love or link with,/The anesthetic from which none come round" (Larkin 1977). This permanent lack of sentience and ability to interact with others is true of the brain-dead patient as well as the corpse. Whereas death is the irreversible end of life, brain death is the irreversible end of the experience that makes life valuable. Brain-dead individuals are, and will remain, experientially dead to the world, though still biologically inter-acting with the world so as to sustain life, with the aid of medical technology and nursing care. (We speak of people who are sleeping also as dead to the world, but they certainly are not as good as dead because they are expected to awake or can be awakened.) Brain-dead patients are objectively alive but subjectively dead—their experiential life is over—making them as good as dead. Having no chance of recovering consciousness, brain-dead individuals have no interests that are set back and thus no harm or wrong done by ending their lives or by procuring their organs, with valid consent, while they remain on life support.

Individuals can also be as good as dead by virtue of their *trajectory*. Those individuals with plans to withdraw LST are as good as dead when their death is imminent and they are at a point of no return along a trajectory to procuring their vital organs prior or subsequent to stopping LST. It is important to be careful how this trajectory is specified. Consider once again the situation of a patient with high-level cervical quadriplegia who has made an autonomous decision to stop mechanical ventilation and donate their organs before dying. We have argued that no harm will come to such a person if vital organs are procured, under conditions of adequate anesthesia, prior to stopping LST. At the time that organs are about to be procured, this still living, but anesthe-tized, individual is now as good as dead. He is on a trajectory that with or without organ procurement, would imminently lead to his becoming dead by stopping mechanical ventilation, making it permissible to retrieve vital organs before stopping treatment. Certainly, this person would not be as good as dead prior to, or even at the time of, his decision to stop LST. He might have made the decision a month before the planned treatment withdrawal, in order to provide ample time to take care of unfinished business. He might in the intervening period change his mind. It clearly would be wrong for another to kill him on the rationale that now that he has made the decision to end his life he has become as good as dead. For there is value in his continued living until the time of planned withdrawal of life support, and, moreover, he did not authorize the other to kill him. But at the point of being anesthetized for the purpose of procuring vital organs, conditional on the patient's prior decision to stop LST, it now makes sense to describe his situation as being as good as dead. Such donors on life support are not yet dead but unalterably will become dead in a very short period of time, and they, or their surrogates, have authorized organ procurement prior to death.

Almost everyone judges it appropriate to procure vital organs for transplan-tation, with valid consent, from dead bodies. We have argued that this is also appropriate for those individuals who are "brain dead" and for those with prior plans to withdraw LST. Their being as good as dead, by virtue of status or trajectory, is equivalent to their being in a situation in which, though still living, they are not harmed or wronged by having vital organs procured. Being as good as dead makes it permissible to operate to retrieve their vital organs before they are dead, just as it is permissible to procure vital organs from dead bodies. These individuals have no need for their organs, so that nothing is lost and something of great potential is gained by transplanting their organs in the bodies of those who need them to survive.

Some might object that individuals who satisfy the clinical criteria for a diagnosis of brain death are not as good as dead (by virtue of their status) because absolute certainty is lacking that they entirely lack the capacity for consciousness, or because they remain alive and their life, though profoundly compromised, deserves respect. However, to support vital organ donation from still-living but "brain-dead" donors, it is not necessary to insist that they are as good as dead by virtue of their status. If their neurological status does not necessarily make them as good as dead, they still are as good as dead with respect to their trajectory, given valid decisions to withdraw LST and donate organs.

The difference between being dead and being as good as dead can be understood as follows. We have argued that to be dead is to be in a condition defined biologically—the irreversible cessation of the functioning of the organism as a whole. Given a biological definition of death, to be dead is a matter of fact, ascertainable by ordinary observation or medical expertise. To be as good as dead is to be in a condition defined normatively—that is, individuals who are alive but as good as dead will not be harmed or wronged if, in some respects, they are treated as if they were dead. There are good reasons for treating individuals in specified circumstances as being as good as dead despite remaining alive. To be sure, not everyone will accept the concept of being as good as dead. Some will see an unbridgeable moral gulf between appropriate treatment of individuals who are alive and bodies that are dead, which leaves no moral space for individuals who are alive but as good as dead. According to this view, interventions that are appropriate for dead bodies, such as vital organ harvesting, can never be appropriate for living human beings. Although not irrational, this vitalistic perspective would imply drastic curtailment of vital organ transplantation if we are right that "brain-dead" individuals remain alive and donors under DCDD protocols are not known to be dead.

The phrase "as good as dead" not only harmonizes with our ethical framework for vital organ donation, it also accurately characterizes the status quo, despite the fact that this is not acknowledged. "Brain-dead" donors are not dead, and donors under DCDD protocols are not known to be dead. Although treated in clinical practice and by the law as dead at the time their organs are removed for transplantation, these donors are as good as dead. In other words, the justification of vital organ donation, in order to be coherent with the established biological conception of death, depends on regarding the donors not as dead but as good as dead. The conceptual error that underlies our current normative perspective on vital organ donation is conflating still-living donors, who are as good as dead, with those who really are dead. The biological conception of death has been fudged to encompass those who are as good as dead in order to pave the way to vital organ transplantation without violating the DDR. In this chapter we have provided and defended an ethical rationale for vital organ transplantation that avoids fictions or fudging the truth regarding the determination of death and thus forthrightly abandons the DDR. In Chapter 7 we will discuss a pragmatic compromise approach to vital organ donation that preserves the DDR by relying on transparent legal fictions relating to the determination of death.

PRACTICAL CONSIDERATIONS

It is incumbent on us to face the practical difficulties posed by our ethical account of vital organ donation without the DDR. The task is daunting. However, we suggest that those who favor the status quo are not entitled to take comfort in the inertia that favors "business as usual" or in the maxim that "if it ain't broke don't fix it" (Capron 1999). We have argued that our current practices of vital organ donation violate the DDR. Patients diagnosed as "brain dead" are not biologically dead, in view of the range of vital functioning they can sustain with the aid of mechanical ventilation. Patients whose organs are extracted a very short interval after asystole are on the verge of death, but we can't be justified in declaring them dead because the cessation of cardiac function might be reversible by resuscitative efforts. It follows that transplant clinicians are routinely procuring vital organs from still-living patients. If we are right about this, then the prevailing ethical defense of the status quo, based on the DDR, is bankrupt. If transplantation of vital organs is to continue, it is necessary to search for an alternative ethical justification of vital organ donation, as we have strived to do. Nonetheless, it is possible that all things considered, it will be necessary to continue to muddle through by endorsing the DDR as an ethical and legal requirement despite the fact that our current practices violate it. This means that we are justifying our practices on the basis of moral and legal fictions. The appeal to fictions can, at best, be an unsatisfactory compromise, which we discuss in Chapter 7. Accordingly, it is important to assess the practical implications of an open policy of vital organ donation without the DDR, with an eye to the prospects for coming to grips honestly with the reality of organ transplantation.

Abandoning the DDR poses serious practical concerns that must be addressed. Will the trust in the medical profession that underwrites the practice of organ donation be eroded if the public believes that organ donors are not dead at the time that vital organs are procured for transplantation? Will transplant surgeons and supporting clinicians be prepared to procure vital organs from patient-donors recognized as still living? When vital organ donation is recognized as extracting organs from still-living patients, how will transplant surgeons escape liability for homicide?

It is facile to presume a public backlash to vital organ transplantation without the DDR. Whether, however, adherence to the DDR is necessary to maintain public trust in the practice of organ donation is an empirical issue. It is not clear that most people believe that brain death constitutes death; however, we doubt that many lay people have given any thought to whether patients should be regarded as dead within a few minutes after their hearts have stopped beating in order to proceed with organ donation. In Chapter 3 we discussed evidence that clinicians have doubts as to whether a diagnosis of brain death constitutes death. If clinicians who are educated about brain death harbor such doubts, there is all the more reason to suspect that the public is not convinced that those declared dead on the basis of neurological criteria are in fact dead. News articles frequently describe brain death as a condition distinct from death (Truog 2007). For example, a recent report of a policeman killed in the line of duty stated that "A police officer shot during a traffic stop was pronounced brain-dead but remained on life support. . . . Oakland police spokesman Jeff Thomason . . . said that [officer] Hege was being kept alive while a final decision was made about donating his organs" (Collins and Leff 2009). Such reports may reflect the way that members of the public view these cases; and it is noteworthy that they do not generate outrage that patients are being killed to procure organs for transplantation. The public may be prepared to see the brain dead as "as good as dead," thus legitimating vital organ donation from living patients.

Survey data are ambiguous with respect to public attitudes relating to the DDR. A telephone survey of a randomly selected sample of 1350 adults in Ohio found that "significant numbers of people were willing to donate the organs of patients they had classified as alive" (Siminoff et al. 2004, 2331). Surveys designed to probe this issue more systematically would be desirable prior to any effort to formally abandon the DDR. Additionally, public education would be a necessary condition for any successful policy change. In sum, this practical concern relating to public trust does not obviously amount to an insurmountable barrier.

The voices of family members who have faced decisions to donate vital organs under tragic circumstances also deserve consideration in assessing public attitudes. In the case of a child who donated organs through a DCDD protocol, for example, the parents stated that if they had found out that another child had died because they were not able to donate their daughter's heart, it would have been "like another slap in our faces." Indeed, they would have permitted simply taking out their daughter's heart under general anesthesia— without the choreographed process of stopping life support, waiting for a short period of time before declaring death, and then intervening to procure organs for transplantation. When pressed about the fact that this would have violated the DDR, the father replied, "There was no chance at all that our daughter was going to survive. . . I can follow the ethicist's argument, but it seems totally ludicrous" (Sanghavi 2009). Although this statement reflects only a single anecdote, it suggests that members of the public can accept as reasonable procuring organs from imminently dying patients prior to stopping life support.

We submit that our ethical justification of vital organ donation accords with common sense and therefore would not be difficult for members of the public to comprehend and endorse. It is not difficult to appreciate that patients who meet the clinical criteria for "brain death" are permanently unconscious and thus have no prospect of return to any meaningful life. Likewise, it is easy to see that patients will die after withdrawing LST, whether this is understood as allowing them to die or causing their death. Procuring vital organs prior to implementing the plan of withdrawing LST does not change the outcome for these patients and offers the opportunity for viable life-saving transplantation, which in fact is not possible in the case of donors who are known to be dead. Nearly everyone recognizes justified cases of killing, and it is not unreasonable to anticipate that most people would see the causing of death involved in the process of procuring vital organs in the context of a prior plan to withdraw LST as ethically appropriate. Finally, requiring consent for both treatment withdrawal and organ donation will reassure the public that vulnerable patients are not being exploited for the good of others. As we have indicated above, we recognize that universal agreement with this ethical framework is not to be expected. Those who endorse strict positions relating to the sanctity of human life, including adherents of Catholic moral theology or many orthodox Jews, will likely oppose interventions to procure vital organs from patients understood as still living; indeed, the latter are often opposed to withdrawing LST, though they regard withholding treatment that is not considered beneficial for the patient as legitimate (Ravitsky 2005). Nevertheless, in a liberal democracy, public policy supported by the law permits practices that some find deeply objectionable.

Clinicians may have more difficulty, at least initially, in accepting our ethical framework for justifying vital organ donation, despite the argument that procuring vital organs from still-living patients on life support is compatible with professional integrity. The framework relies on understanding withdrawal of LST as causing death. However, as we discussed in Chapter 1, conventional medical ethics regards treatment withdrawal as merely allowing patients to die from their underlying medical condition. The traditional prohibition on intentional killing of patients, which prohibits active euthanasia by administering lethal medication, is likely to be seen as also prohibiting procuring vital organs from living patients. On the other hand, a basic factual premise that gives rise to the need for justifying vital organ donation without appeal to the DDR is that current practices, nominally governed by the DDR, are procuring vital organs from patients who are not dead. This premise relies on the established definition of death recognized within medicine in terms of the irreversible cessation of the functioning of the organism as a whole. Attention to the incompatibility between this definition of death and current transplantation practices should foster openness to an alternative ethical justification, especially as transplant clinicians dedicated to saving the lives of desperately ill patients will be averse to abandoning the procurement of vital organs. Educational efforts should help in promoting acceptance of vital organ donation without the DDR.

Concerns about exposing transplant surgeons to legal liability for homicide by virtue of procuring vital organs from still-living patients appear to pose a more formidable practical challenge. Even if some clinicians are prepared to risk liability, it is doubtful that the courts would declare vital organ procurement that results in a patient's death as outside the scope of criminal homicide. Alternatively, changing homicide laws would be a difficult undertaking. Dramatic legal change of this sort is not impossible, as legislation was passed throughout the United States, within a relatively short period of time, to recognize the legality of declaring death on the basis of neurological criteria. This legal transformation occurred with very little controversy. In contrast, a proposal to change the homicide laws to accommodate vital organ donation from living patients is apt to be highly controversial, especially in view of the "culture wars" and intense partisanship that have characterized social policy in the United States in recent years.

FINAL OBJECTION

We come now to a final objection that we can imagine a critic making to our account of vital organ donation, and to other arguments in the book that challenge conventional medical ethics. "Why are you stirring up trouble? Let's grant that you are right that the established ethical perspective on organ transplantation relies on a fiction that those diagnosed as 'brain dead' are dead and on fudging the truth about those declared dead under DCDD protocols. So what?

Since the beginning of vital organ transplantation, clinicians, family members of donors, and the general public have found moral comfort in the conviction, or at least the official view, that vital organs are being procured only from the dead. You should let sleeping dogs lie. A radical proposal such as abandoning the DDR risks imperiling the life-saving enterprise of transplantation."

We take this objection seriously. In reply, we note that controversy over the determination of death as it relates to organ donation has characterized the scholarly literature over the past 20 years (Truog 1997; Shewmon 1998). There is nothing new in our insistence that current practices, in fact, violate the DDR. Yet established medical ethics has remained impervious to the facts about vital organ donation. Because honesty and commitment to the truth are values of great importance, ethical frameworks that rely on fictions and fudges are inherently suspect. Similarly, public policies in a democracy, committed to rational discussion, should be defensible without reliance on falsehood. And no policies, no matter how entrenched, should be immune from criticism. We would reluctantly agree with this critic's admonition if we thought there were no prospect of acceptance by clinicians and the public of a sound alternative ethical framework. In any case, we judge it highly unlikely that vigorous scholarly criticism of the prevailing medical ethics relating to organ donation or withdrawing LST will undermine these widely accepted practices. It may eventually, however, contribute to reconstructing medical ethics on a foundation that does not rely on fictions and fudges and morally biased judgments of fact.

MUDDLING THROUGH

Regardless of what is ideal and desirable in the long run, we face the question of how to proceed here and now. Current practices of vital organ donation, as a matter of fact, violate the DDR. This fact is masked by appeal to moral fictions regarding the status of living, or not clearly dead, bodies from which vital organs are currently being procured (Miller et al. 2010). Despite growing awareness and professional discussion regarding the incoherence between theory and practice in this domain, the DDR appears to remain an unshakeable moral and legal norm. Brock (1999) has argued that in making and discussing public policy we sometimes face choices between "truth or consequences." If the consequences of abandoning the dubious determinations of death supporting our current practices of organ transplantation and the DDR would be to undermine public confidence and thus reduce the supply of organs, then it would be better to maintain the moral status quo. Consequences would trump the truth. We have our doubts that these deleterious consequences would necessarily ensue from honestly facing the reality of our current practices of vital organ donation.

Nevertheless, the difficulty in effecting the legal change relating to criminal homicide necessary to formally abandon the DDR would seem to make it unlikely that this will happen any time soon.

Once we recognize the fictions underlying the status quo, it becomes difficult to pay lip service to the DDR as a moral norm. Is there any way to maintain honesty and intellectual integrity in face of the conceptual incoherence that characterizes the practice of vital organ donation today? In Chapter 7 we discuss a practical alternative to the status quo of organ transplantation that relies on the concept of legal fictions.

7

Legal Fictions Approach to Organ Donation, with Seema K. Shah

We closed the last chapter with the recognition that abandoning the dead donor rule (DDR) poses practical difficulties that make it unrealistic to expect that the alternative ethical account for vital organ donation that we recommend has the prospect of gaining wide support and becoming institutionalized in the near future. In the meantime, is there a way to make progress within the current legal framework that endorses the DDR, a neurological criterion for determining death, and practices of donation after circulatory determination of death (DCDD)? In this chapter, we argue that current practices when viewed in light of facts relating to vital organ donation are based on a set of *unacknowledged* legal fictions. We argue further that a process of transforming these unacknowledged legal fictions into transparent legal fictions permits recognition of the fact that vital organs are being procured from donors who are not dead or not known to be dead without overturning established legal norms. Although this legal fictions approach is far from ideal, it may be the best that can be achieved in the short run and may become the catalyst for ethical and legal reconstruction that more honestly faces the truth about vital organ donation.

ARE OUR STANDARDS FOR DETERMINING DEATH FICTIONS?

Does the determination of death in the context of current practices of vital organ donation involve legal fictions? To answer this question, we must first understand what legal fictions are and what they are not.

Defining Legal Fictions

Fictions pervade many aspects of life. Fictions are untruths, whether patently false or not, that are treated as true and used in the service of particular ends. They may be benign attempts to appease social or other concerns, or may be used to avoid the cognitive dissonance of noticing that two practices do not fit together, even though it is not desirable to abandon either. At the most super-ficial level, fictions are commonly employed to maintain social harmony, as when you compliment a host for a "delicious" dinner that was not very good, or when to ease the worries of people who think the number 13 is unlucky, hotels simply refer to the 13th floor as the the "14th" floor (Bix 2009). On an individual level, there is empirical evidence that subjects will create fictions for themselves in order to resolve cognitive dissonance (Festinger and Carlsmith 1959). Fictions also operate on much larger levels, when we as a society would rather not confront the dissonance between two dearly held beliefs, such as the fiction that judges merely act as "umpires" who strive to implement the rules they are given, as opposed to political and fundamentally human actors who really do shape the law and even create new law in certain cases (Frank 1973).

Legal fictions are a special category of fiction. Although legal fictions have been defined in different ways by legal scholars, Lon Fuller's classic book gives perhaps the clearest and most thorough account of legal fictions (Fuller 1967). A legal fiction is essentially a metaphorical or heuristic device that involves making a clearly false statement or claim in order to serve some legal purpose. A legal fiction can be "either (1) a statement propounded with a complete or partial consciousness of its falsity, or (2) a false statement recognized as having utility" (Fuller 1967, 9). Legal fictions are not intended to deceive, but rather to allow the law to expand into new areas while tempering the degree of change that the law must undergo. There may be times when the law must accommo-date new concepts, and fictions are the "growing pains" of the law. They may be especially important in cases in which it is not clear how the law can best address a novel situation. The classic example of a legal fiction is the fact that the law *treats* corporations as persons, even though it is perfectly clear that a corpora-tion is different from what we usually consider is a person. Judges do not attempt to hide the fact that a corporation is different from a person in many ways, but treating corporations as persons allows judges to know what to do with corpo-rations, because they fit into a legal category that has already been established.

Legal fictions may develop gradually. For instance, multiple courts may be involved in developing a fiction over time—one court can start the work, and others can build on that precedent to allow the law to grow in a particular direc-tion. As the history of the determination of death illustrates, respected scientific bodies may issue recommendations that the law later follows. Without the ability to assess the scientific validity of those recommendations, lawmakers may be led astray and may codify a legal approach that does not reflect the facts. The fictive nature of law may also become evident over time. For instance, laws may be created based on an understanding that a certain factual claim is true, and advancing empirical evidence may, over time, transform that law into a legal fiction. Alternatively, practice in a given field may advance beyond what the existing law permits, but legal authorities may see no need to reconcile the law and practice overtly, thereby allowing the reconciliation of the two to be done by a fiction instead. Fictions that form in this manner include the determination of death for the purpose of organ transplantation, which we will discuss in the next two sections. These fictions are likely to be unacknowledged and opaque (Fuller 1967, 8).

Does "Whole Brain Death" Count as a Legal Fiction?

The idea that brain death is a legal fiction has been explicitly rejected by two U.S. public bioethics commissions that have developed reports on the determination of death based on a biological definition. The President's Commission was careful to describe their policy recommendation to adopt the whole brain criterion for determining death as one that "must accurately reflect the social meaning of death and not constitute a mere legal fiction" (President's Commission 1981, 31). Twenty seven years (and much controversy) later, the President's Council argued for the need to develop a new biological rationale for "total brain failure" as a criterion for determining death, owing to the recognition that patients diagnosed as "brain dead" may continue to manifest a range of integrative functioning of the organism as a whole with the aid of mechanical ventilation. Even so, they emphasized that the definition of death as total brain failure should *not* be thought of as a legal construct in order to promote organ donation. Instead, they claimed that the neurological standard for determining death is scientifically sufficient to reach an accurate conclusion that death has occurred (President's Council 2008, 50, 130).

Although we do not regard these two commission reports as disingenuous about "brain death" not being a legal fiction, the way in which they both summarily rejected this way of understanding the neurological criterion for determining death seems suspect. It appears from these disclaimers that these two public bioethics commissions did not think that a legal fiction approach could be legitimate, but implicitly acknowledged that there are reasons to think that the whole brain criterion might be a legal fiction. As discussed in Chapter 3, many critics have questioned whether individuals can be truly dead when they have sustained neurological injury consistent with a diagnosis of "brain death" but continue to circulate blood, breathe, and perform other biological functions with the aid of mechanical ventilation. These strong denunciations by public bioethics commissions suggest that if the whole brain criterion is a legal fiction, it is unacknowledged.

Alta Charo has argued that the definition of death is a legal fiction because she thinks death is an ambiguous concept, and any line we draw will not accurately capture all of the relevant cases (Charo 1999). This type of fiction involves "bright line" rules that are designed to capture most, but perhaps not all, cases. One example of this type of fiction is the rule that after a person has been missing for 7 years, that person is declared legally dead. It may be a reasonable assumption that a person who has been missing for 7 years is in fact dead, but there is no way to be certain about every case. Nevertheless, this approach allows assets to be divided up and used by others and allows surviving spouses to remarry, thus resulting in an outcome that is better than continuous uncertainty in most cases. Another example is the classification "legally blind," which creates a defined legal category for people who qualify as eligible for assistance or services based on their vision falling below a certain threshold, even though they may actually retain some sight. Yet another example is how the rights and responsibilities of adulthood are granted to individuals. As soon as a child turns 18, that child is legally transformed into an adult, with rights to do things such as vote, marry without parental permission, and consent for contracts, medical treatment, or participation in research. Yet children do not magically become adults when they turn 18. Each individual person grows and matures at different rates, and some children are more mature than many adults. It would be unworkable to have completely different standards for adulthood for every person, depending on his or her personal maturity and competency. Rather, the law draws a bright line that sometimes gets it right, but can be both under- and overinclusive.

Bright line fictions will often track the truth, and they would be unreasonable if they mostly failed to do so. Their falsity comes from the claim that the bright line demarcates the correct distinction in all cases. With respect to adulthood, for instance, the bright line drawn at the age of 18 fails to consider some adolescents adults even when they are ready for the rights and responsibilities that would result, and it also fails to distinguish adults who are slower to mature than others and gives them rights and responsibilities for which they may be ill-prepared. These types of fictions make it easier to draft laws when there are a variety of different cases the law has to cover—they increase the law's ability to dispatch complex cases without requiring a great deal of judicial reasoning. They also do a better job of providing clear notice to people about how the law will treat a particular issue than a case-by-case approach would.

Do the determinations of death in contemporary medicine reflect bright line fictions that allow for administrability in the judicial process, as Charo suggests? It may be that death is very difficult to define, and creating a rule to define death that can be administered consistently across the land is nearly impossible. If that was true, there may be legitimate reasons for turning to a legal fiction instead of throwing our hands up and merely stating that death is very difficult, if not impossible, to define. Yet the whole brain criterion for determining death is not a bright line rule that fails to capture all relevant cases. The commissions that have endorsed the determination of death based on a diagnosis of "brain death" have defended it on the grounds that it captures the truth about death, not that it captures some but not all cases. In addition, the fact that some states allow for different definitions of death for people of different religious faiths suggests that the need for one consistent bright line rule is hardly paramount (Olick et al. 2009). Finally, the traditional and common-sense understanding of death is that death occurs when the functions of the heart and lung have ceased and they cannot be resuscitated—when a person becomes a corpse. This appears to be a relatively easy and clear way to define death, which is fully suitable for most legal purposes, so it is unlikely that the administrability concerns alone are what motivated this fiction. It has to be something else—the drive for organ donation—that has led medicine and the law away from the default, traditional criteria for determining death.

Because whole-brain death is simply not the same as death, understood in accordance with the established biological conception, this legal fiction is better described as a "status fiction" that draws an analogy between two clearly different concepts. Status fictions, like the fiction that a corporation is a person, are fictions that treat A *as if* it were B because they are relevantly similar for determining what law should apply to them. Whole-brain death does not fit with the biological definition of death established in medical practice and endorsed by public bioethics commissions or with the common concept of death. It is a state in which profound neurological damage causes the permanent loss of consciousness, which arguably makes people's lives lacking in any humanly significant value; but it strains credibility to think that a corpse can remain warm to the touch, heal wounds, gestate babies, or go through puberty. In sum, the whole-brain criterion of death is not a bright line fiction that captures some cases and not others. Rather, it is a "status" legal fiction that permits us to treat individuals who are not dead as if they are dead.

Standard "status" fictions that are legal fictions are transparent fictions. No one actually thinks that a corporation is a person similar to a human being. By contrast, it is simply not true that everyone knows that whole-brain death is not death. Because it lacks transparency, it seems that the whole-brain standard of death is best understood as an *unacknowledged* legal fiction—one that conceals the normative choice that it is permissible to procure vital organs from individuals with profound neurological damage and no chance of recovery who in fact remain alive. Those who are not dead are treated as if they are dead for the purpose of organ donation without any general recognition that this is occurring. When the whole-brain death criterion was first introduced, it is possible that it may have been developed and maintained because of concerns about the legitimacy of organ donation, without much attention to why the condition of profound neurological injury involving irreversible apneic coma constitutes death. In any case, as discussed in Chapter 3, it was believed that cessation of circulatory functioning would inevitably and quickly follow the diagnosis of brain death regardless of technological interventions. Today, however, the evidence is in, and it is clear that whole-brain death is not death on the basis of a biological definition relating to the functioning of the organism as a whole.

Some might argue that there are important moral reasons for maintaining but not acknowledging this fiction, that it is necessary to allow the practice of organ donation to have legitimacy in the eyes of the public. If organ donation would not be politically feasible without the public being deceived about when death occurs, then there may be substantial reasons behind the existence and maintenance of this unacknowledged legal fiction, but also considerable dangers. The claim may be that achieving this important end requires deceiving the public, but without empirical evidence to support this claim, it is problematic that such a value-laden and important issue remains outside the realm of issues on which we have public and democratic deliberation.

Does DCDD Involve a Legal Fiction?

The determination of death in the context of DCDD protocols involves a different type of legal fiction, but one that is also unacknowledged. The legal fiction operating in DCDD derives from fudging the meaning of the word "irreversibility." DCDD requires that a person's circulatory function stops irreversibly. However, donors are declared dead according to circulatory–respiratory criteria when there is at least some, and perhaps significant, uncertainty about the irreversibility of the loss of circulatory function. Because physicians are procuring vital organs shortly after asystole, when it is possible, though unlikely, that circulation might be restored spontaneously and likely that resuscitative measures could be successful in restoring circulation, especially when the heart is removed and can be restarted in another person, there will be at least some cases in which death is determined prematurely. To obviate this, doctors could wait longer to make the determination, but this would entail a significant cost in terms of lives that could be saved by organ donation.

As discussed in Chapter 5, some commentators have proposed that in the context of DCDD, however, irreversibility should be understood differently. Instead of asking whether there was any possibility that the heart could have been restarted if doctors used all life-saving measures, we should focus on the limits of what doctors can legally do in these situations. Because doctors cannot legally force life-saving measures on a person who has decided to stop treatment or refuse attempts at resuscitation, and because doing so would be unethical and a violation of that person's autonomy, a determination of death on circulatory criteria under these circumstances reflects normative irreversibility.

We have argued that this approach fudges the normal meaning of "irreversibility"—what is not possible to reverse by available means, rather than what might be reversible but would be wrong to attempt. However, the circumstances under which organs are procured following withdrawal of life support is one in which it seems reasonable to treat the dying person as if he or she was already dead. The determination of death in DCDD cases involves what we would call an "anticipatory fiction." An anticipatory fiction is a fiction that allows an event to be treated as if it has occurred, even though it has not, because it will imminently occur and waiting for it to happen will result in harm. Therefore, we are justified in treating something as if that state has been reached, even before it actually has. For example, a person can be held in breach of contract even before the deadline for performance has passed if they have not yet fulfilled the terms of the contract, but it becomes unequivocally clear that they will be unable or unwilling to do so in time (*Combs v. Int'l Ins. Co.* 2004). This is known as anticipatory breach. In contract law, the court draws a firm line that the anticipated breach be unequivocal or absolute. This may be important to ensure that the standard for anticipatory breach does not drift too far in the direction of permitting lawsuits for breaches that may or may not occur. Another example is the use of declaratory judgments to prevent patent holders from using their patents as "scarecrows" in an attempt to protect intellectual territory. Federal courts are generally not permitted to issue advisory opinions on abstract legal questions, and have to address real controversies. To protect the rights of an inventor who has developed a device (or is about to), and is legitimately concerned about infringing a patent, however, courts do not force these inventors to wait until they are sued for patent infringement. Instead, they allow inventors to bring suit for declaratory judgments if they reasonably suspect that a patent owner would sue them if they continued to do work on their invention (Munsell 1997).

Many have argued that we know for certain that a person's heart and circulation will not spontaneously restart 20 minutes after asystole (provided that the body has not been maintained at a low temperature) (Machado and Korein 2009). Furthermore, some European protocols for DCDD wait 10 minutes after asystole (Sanchez-Fructuouso et al. 2006). But even setting aside the issue of whether cardiopulmonary resuscitation (CPR) might have been successful in restoring circulation, 2 minutes is likely not sufficient to be completely certain that death has occurred, especially when certain organ-preserving measures may have the unintended effect of reviving the heart. Waiting longer amounts of time might fail to respect the wishes of people who wanted to donate their organs and compromise the success of organ transplantation, or even render it impossible. To justify the trade-off being made here, a legal fiction is being employed—the idea that because individuals are on the verge of death (with no permissible means of averting it), and waiting until they are known to be dead would cause harm, we can treat them as if they were dead. Importantly, there are no legal duties that prevent doctors from being able to rely on this fiction. Doctors in this situation do not have a duty to attempt to resuscitate the person; in fact, they legally cannot and ethically should not do so. Moreover, the patient/donor and/or the family have already given consent to organ donation. These protections help minimize the risk that this anticipatory legal fiction will run roughshod over other legal duties.

MOVING TO TRANSPARENT LEGAL FICTIONS

The unacknowledged legal fictions underlying contemporary determinations of death in the context of organ procurement are problematic because they divert attention from and distort the truth about important, life-saving practices. Perhaps the most plausible and least disruptive solution for the short term is to endeavor to transform these unacknowledged legal fictions into transparent legal fictions. This would allow the law to permit vital organ transplantation to continue with organs donated by individuals who are regarded as legally dead despite remaining biologically alive or not known with certainty to be dead.

Thus, the determination that patients diagnosed with "total brain failure" are dead and the declaration of death in DCDD protocols might be seen as (transparent) fictions to facilitate life-saving organ donation without formally abandoning the DDR, revising conventional medical ethics, and changing the law relating to homicide. Of course, standard legal fictions are transparent and evident and those who use them should be aware of their limitations. The public and clinicians do not clearly understand that the determination of death on the basis of total brain failure treats still-living individuals with permanent loss of consciousness as if they were dead. It should be clear that the legal standards for determining death do not, in all respects, track the truth of the matter. Turning the determinations of death in the context of organ donation into legitimate, transparent legal fictions will require an evolution in awareness by the professions and the public. This would require openness about the purposes the legal but fictive determination of death serves in this context and the ways in which it may depart from biological reality.

Practically speaking, a change such as this might begin with the legal and medical professions and bioethics scholars. The literature and professional practice should reflect the truth about death by using legal fictions terminology. This might be most notable in the way professionals and courts talk about death as whole-brain death. Instead of describing a person as dead, they would note that once a person has been diagnosed with total brain failure, the law will treat that person as if he or she were dead. As this transparent legal fictions approach spreads, the news media is likely to reflect this change and begin reporting whole-brain death and DCDD as legal fictions. People would come to recognize that being legally dead is not the same as being biologically dead. It is possible that some more systematic approach to public education would ultimately be required. One suggestion we would make is that a future bioethics commission should help to clarify the confusion that previous bioethics commissions have helped to create. Given that prior bioethics commissions have contributed to the creation of unacknowledged legal fictions about death, all the while denying that they were talking about legal fictions, a new bioethics commission may bear some obligation to set the record straight. At the very least, such a commission should discuss seriously the merits of a legal fictions strategy instead of summarily dismissing this approach.

This increased transparency would also have to extend to the consent for donation given by patients and their families. Patients, families, and the public would have to understand that a diagnosis of "total brain failure" is not actually death, but that it counts as being legally dead and makes vital organ donation appropriate because it is a state in which there is no chance of recovery of consciousness and the ability to interact with others. It may make sense to give people different options for organ donation based on circumstances that they may find themselves in. Organ donor cards could have checkboxes that have options in which some people would elect to have their organs donated only if they had experienced total brain failure, and others would like to donate their organs only if a certain amount of time had passed after the cessation of circulatory function. Because of its increased transparency, this use of a legal fiction, once it becomes widely understood, does not raise significant concerns about subverting democratic deliberation or obtaining organs from people without their informed consent, concerns that are clearly raised by the current use of an unacknowledged legal fiction.

Our hope is that this legal fictions approach may serve as a necessary inter-mediate step to allow the law to move forward, or function as "scaffolding" for the law (Fuller 1967, 70). For instance, in Ancient Rome, foreigners were initially not subject to Roman law. To integrate foreigners into society and ensure that lawlessness was not encouraged by the presence of noncitizens, judges were instructed to treat foreigners as if they were citizens. What was notable is that this legal fiction was out in the open, and created a transparent solution in which the law applied to foreigners and citizens alike (Harmon 1990, 13). In Rome, the scaffolding provided adequate support for the law to grow in a new and important direction, and this would hopefully be true of legal fictions used in the determination of death context today, if these fictions are acknowledged.

Like a move toward complete transparency, treating the determination of death in the context of vital organ donation and the dead donor rule as legal fictions is not without costs. This approach could undermine social support for termination of life support and organ donation for people who have experi-enced total brain failure. One interesting thing to note here is that the public is comfortable with legal fictions, and several legal fictions are widely known to be untrue (or are patently false). The public also seems able to distinguish brain death from death, and appears, to a large extent, to treat these two categories differently (Dubois and Schmidt 2003). These facts provide some reassurance that the fear of significant costs as a result of using a legal fiction may not mate-rialize. The social processes that would be involved in this transformation may have already begun. Scholars, journalists, and clinicians have begun to describe the brain-death criterion in ways that suggest a movement from an unacknowl-edged to a transparent legal fiction. As awareness and transparency of its status as a legal fiction spread, provided that enough consensus builds in the field, eventually the truth underlying this legal fiction may be endorsed by courts and/or legislatures.

Identifying an accurate definition of death that will allow for organ procure-ment from " donors with "total brain failure" seems elusive, but relatively easy, in theory, with respect to DCDD. Erring on the side of caution for DCDD, we could permit organ transplantation only from bodies that are clearly dead by waiting 10–20 minutes before organ procurement to ensure that cessation of circulation has occurred and is irreversible in the strictest sense. This alterna-tive has considerable costs, however, and does not seem warranted. It would inevitably result in significant loss of organs that could be used to save the lives of others, and would not adequately respect the wishes of those who want to stop receiving treatment and to donate their organs to others.

Moreover, because there is a plausible legal interpretation of "irreversibility" that could justify physicians waiting fewer than 10–20 minutes after asystole, it is not clear that this cautious approach is legally required. Once again, there is a fiction involved here because legal irreversibility does not coincide with irreversibility in fact. Use of this fiction to permit retrieving organs shortly after asystole, when they are more likely to be viable, is ethically justifiable. Under DCDD protocols, within a few minutes after their hearts have stopped beating patient-donors are on a trajectory of no return to imminent death. Although resuscitative measures might be successful in restoring circulation, making it unclear whether they are actually dead at the time they are declared dead, they or their families have made valid prior decisions to both refuse treatment and CPR. In this situation, we have argued that they have no interests that would be set back by procuring vital organs in anticipation of their death, making them as good as dead. People who have decided that they retain no interest in remaining alive, would like their therapy to be stopped, and who do have an interest in donating their organs cannot be harmed by allowing their organs to be harvested. Of course, there may be some other potential harms to consider, such as whether organ removal from people who are not dead would cause suffering. However, the risks of this harm could easily be minimized, if not eliminated, by the use of analgesics and anesthesia. Notwithstanding the fact that people who donate organs under these circumstances are neither harmed nor wronged, current practices of DCDD do rely on an unacknowledged anticipatory legal fiction. The argument for making this legal fiction transparent in the case of brain death also holds for DCDD.

One open question is whether the current approach of using an anticipatory legal fiction could justify removing organs in even shorter periods of time after asystole (or even no time at all) for controlled and/or uncontrolled DCDD. It is possible that the current approach could eventually lead to withdrawing organs from people who have not been declared dead under circulatory criteria, but who do not wish further treatment and do wish to donate their organs. Although this progression is justifiable on ethical grounds, as argued in Chapter 6, there may be good reasons to draw a line that prevents us from reaching this destination by means of relying on the anticipatory legal fiction alone. Through a process of democratic deliberation, we may reach a point at which the dead donor rule no longer seems necessary. We are not there yet, however, and a legal fiction should not be employed to conceal such a dramatic, important, and value-laden policy decision. It seems important to reach the outcome of allowing organ donation from those who have made the choice to withdraw or refuse treatment and the choice to donate before treatment withdrawal in an open and forthright manner, which a legal fiction approach could not fully accomplish. Nevertheless, the legal fictions approach that we recommend preserves the dead donor rule as a legal norm that is, to a great extent, fictive in its application—not as a factual requirement of death as a precondition for vital organ donation.

OBJECTIONS TO OUR PROPOSAL

It is important to emphasize that acknowledging these legal fictions is a justifiable policy only if there is a sound ethical rationale for procuring vital organs from still-living patients. Otherwise, we would be acknowledging an unjustified distortion of the truth—a disturbing prospect for the law. A legal fictions approach toward brain death has been criticized by Shewmon as "a pseudo-rationale," which he characterizes as "utilitarianism": "'brain death' is a legal fiction invented to legitimize the transplantation of vital organs that would otherwise be wasted" (Shewmon 1997, 42). This would be a pseudo-rationale if the legal fictions approach was intended to give the impression that brain death constitutes death as a matter of fact. Rather, the intent of the approach that we advance is to treat "brain death" as legal death, despite not really constituting death. The rationale for this is, in some sense, utilitarian, in that it underwrites social benefits from vital organ transplantation. But it is not "utilitarian" in the sense of being merely socially expedient without regard to protecting the rights and well-being of vulnerable patients. In other words, we do not think that the harms being visited on some are justified in terms of gains to others. What legitimizes the procuring of vital organs from brain-dead donors is not the legal fiction but the ethical rationale for making use of organs to save the lives of others when doing so poses no harm or wrong to the donor. The legal fiction serves to harmonize the ethically desirable practice of transplantation with existing laws and policies.

In Chapter 6 we presented and defended in detail an alternative ethical account of vital organ donation without the DDR. This ethical account underwrites the legitimacy of the legal fictions approach. Our current practices of procuring vital organs are ethically justifiable not because donors are dead at the time that organs are retrieved but because no harm or wrong is done to the donors in light either of their status as having permanently lost consciousness and/or the prior valid decision to withdraw life-sustaining treatment (LST), provided that valid consent for donation has been obtained. Obtaining an individual's valid consent for organ donation, or a surrogate's substituted judgment, ensures that the individual endorses the end he or she is serving. Hence, the legal fictions approach that we defend is ethically justifiable because it respects the choices of patients or their surrogates and no harm is done to patient-donors under these conditions. The legal fictions approach treats such donors as dead in the eyes of the law, but this does not attempt to make legitimate what would otherwise be illegitimate. Rather, this approach brings the ethically justified practice of vital organ donation into harmony with the law, given the established norms of the dead donor rule and criminal homicide. In other words, because the former norm is difficult to abandon and the latter is difficult to modify, the legal fictions approach constitutes a useful heuristic device to reconcile the facts regarding our current organ procurement practices with the law. Absent the legal fiction, these established legal norms would preclude or greatly curtail the ethically justified practice of vital organ donation.

Some may criticize our legal fictions approach because they view legal fictions pejoratively as merely expedient in addition to seeing them negatively because they are fictions. We have contended that even maintaining the status quo, however, requires relying on unacknowledged legal fictions. Vital organs are being procured from patient-donors who are still living or at least are not known to be dead. This means that an important question before us is: what is the best way for the law to approach this practice in light of the facts regarding the status of vital organ donors? As we have argued, vital organ donation without the dead donor rule is ethically justifiable but would require large-scale legal change, including modifying homicide laws such that transplant surgeons are not liable for criminal homicide by virtue of causing the deaths of patient-donors.

Weighing and balancing the different ways to harmonize the law with ongoing, ethically justifiable clinical practice requires assessing the practical advantages and disadvantages of alternative policy strategies. In assessing various ways of modifying the law, expedience is an entirely relevant consideration. As compared with the leading alternatives—(1) prohibiting or drastically curtailing vital organ transplantation, (2) abandoning the dead donor rule along with other legal changes required to continue vital organ transplantation without fictions, or (3) merely preserving the unacknowledged legal fictions we have now—a transparent legal fictions approach deserves serious consideration as a pragmatic compromise. The third option of upholding the status quo by attempting to muddle through is the path of least resistance. However, it will require increasing duplicity in the face of the growing scholarly literature that is challenging the rationales for determining death in the practice of organ transplantation. Without a doubt, the legal fictions approach is less than ideal. No matter how transparent it becomes, the use of fictions in the law involves at least an element of sleight of hand—the law declares states of affairs to be different than they in fact are. Significantly, however, it is sleight of hand that is out in the open.

Of course, there are some dangers to allowing legal fictions to persist that are important to recognize and address. For instance, Fuller argues that law should be cleansed of fictions as soon as they are no longer necessary because they involve reasoning by analogy that can lead to errors in thinking (Fuller 1967, 70). The problem is that "inaccurate language can so easily change our substantive views about what is natural or what is right" (Bix 2009, 20). Slippery slope concerns may arise when a fiction can be borrowed too easily from one area of the law to another. For instance, Louise Harmon has argued that the idea that a previously competent person's substituted judgment can be determined by courts, particularly without much reference to the person's actual stated wishes, is a legal fiction. She further claims that although it was relatively unproblematic when used to justify transfers of wealth, it has been inappropriately borrowed by other courts to justify organ donation by or sterilization of people who were never competent (Harmon 1990, 63). In her view, legal fictions can be dangerous if they have the potential to encourage other courts to make larger, less justified leaps away from the truth in a context in which that move is more dangerous or problematic (Harmon 1990, 62).

Although legal fictions can be especially useful when they track our common-sense understanding of how to treat a given situation and maintain conceptual consistency and transparency when changing the law is unlikely to happen soon, there are examples of legal fictions distorting the contours of the law in just the way commentators have worried about. In a recent Supreme Court case, *Citizen's United*, the Supreme Court dramatically extended the political rights of corporations. Some have characterized the decision as polarizing and an example of judicial overreaching, whereas others have given it high praise for preventing the government from regulating speech based on the identity of the speaker (Rosen 2010; Dworkin 2010). What has been less discussed is the role that a legal fiction played in allowing the Court to render its opinion (Marcus 2010). We would argue that depending on the relevant theory underlying the first amendment protection of freedom of speech, the existence of the legal fiction made a decision that might otherwise have been difficult to justify seem like a more natural extension of the law.

In *Citizens United*, the Supreme Court addressed the constitutional limitations on regulation of political speech by corporations. The majority opinion in the case often implies that corporations and individual persons should be treated similarly with respect to the regulation of their political speech, notwithstanding the obvious differences between corporations and individuals. The fiction that a corporation is a person is a device or analogy properly used to determine what law to apply to corporations only in circumstances in which the analogy is useful. For example, questions about whether a court has jurisdiction over a corporation can then be resolved in the same way that those questions would be resolved about persons—based on where they live. On the other hand, an executive who mismanaged a corporation and ran it into the ground would never be criminally charged for murdering that corporation.

One important distinction between corporations and people neglected in *Citizens United* is that corporations are owned by shareholders and run by management. When people engage in political speech, we are not worried that their subparts (organs or personalities, as the case may be) will disagree with their stated opinion. Shareholders may have very diverse political views, and their First Amendment interests will not necessarily be served by allowing corporations to speak, because that speech will be mediated through the corporate managers. The dissent also notes that corporations can be owned by people who are not U.S. citizens. Therefore, this decision allows noncitizens who own corporations to be able to contribute to political campaigns. Ordinary noncitizens do not have that privilege. The majority in *Citizens United* does not address these important differences between corporations and people.

Additionally, some reasons for strong First Amendment protection of individual political speech do not completely extend to corporations. For instance, one explanation the Court gives for this ruling is to prevent "censorship to control thought," because "The First Amendment confirms the freedom to think for ourselves." Although corporations may have opinions or corporate cultures, it is more strange to imagine a corporation—not just individuals within that corporation—thinking. Perhaps one approach would be to say that corporations think when they engage in strategic decision-making practices. Even if that were the case, it is not clear that the freedom to fully engage in strategic decision-making practices, including using corporate funds to influence political campaigns, is as worthy of protection as the freedom of thought that each individual needs to participate in a democracy.

The implications of this decision illustrate other problems with extending the legal fiction. The dissent rightly points out that the implications of this ruling could be that corporations should have other political rights, such as the right to vote. At least, the majority's reason should have elucidated a principle that explains when corporate political rights should be extended and when they should not, to avoid the absurd implication that corporations should have the right to vote in elections. This case illustrates that it may be wise to delineate the limits of a legal fiction in relying on it to make changes in the law.

Most legal fictions, although transparent, raise concerns because they take the law one step away from the truth, and could lead the law even further astray in the long run. The correct limits of the fiction need to be clear and each time the fiction is extended this extension should be thought through and justified. Otherwise, an incorrect use of the fiction, like the analogy that a corporation is a person, can distort the law. As one commentator explained,

> The more pervasive and autonomic is the legal fiction ... the more difficult it becomes to overcome the unconscious tendency to regard the fiction as truth. Indeed, it is that very tendency that makes the fiction of corporate legal personhood so useful and enduring.
>
> Thinking and speaking of a "corporation"—an abstraction representing a multitude of complex relationships—as if it were a real person, rather

than speaking and thinking in terms of the Byzantine relationships implicated by anything a corporation "does," is a nearly indispensable simplifying convention. (Brubaker 2005, 759)

Legal fictions that are insufficiently transparent and persist for long periods of time, however, may make it more likely that logical fallacies may begin to pollute our understanding of the concept. Transparency makes legal fictions less of a threat to the coherence of the law because they do not conceal the truth of the matter or the purpose behind the fiction, but it does not eliminate their potential for misuse. If courts recognize that the purpose of the fiction does not apply to a particular case, suspending the fiction is always an option. Yet, even transparent legal fictions can be abused if the analogies that underlie them are extended in a way that subverts or illegitimately transcends the policy context that justifies such legal fictions.

It is our hope that if the existing legal fictions being used in the determination of death are acknowledged, they can give recognition (but not full transparency) to the normative appropriateness of permitting vital organ donation from some classes of patients who in fact are still alive or not known to be dead. When valid consent for donation is provided, no harm or wrong is done to these patient-donors, and life-saving transplantations become possible by procuring vital organs from them. Appeal to transparent legal fictions is useful in preserving the practice of vital organ transplantation without the need to formally abandon the dead donor rule and to change the homicide laws. Moving from the unacknowledged to transparent legal fictions also is desirable in that it promotes bringing the reality of vital organ transplantation into the light of day, instead of concealing the normative choices involved in this practice. Ultimately, it may (and should) be a step in the direction of more honestly facing the ethical justification for vital organ transplantation without any need for nominal appeal to the dead donor rule.

If appropriately constrained, legal fictions may be particularly useful within a pluralistic society such as ours. Within a pluralistic society, different ways of understanding matters of life and death must be tolerated. A transparent legal fictions approach can be seen as one way of understanding the current practice of vital organ donation. Employing a legal fiction about the determination of death permits the law to be coherent. In particular, if we think people's views about death should be accommodated, as New York and New Jersey have done, then we might think that there should be room for different definitions of death by religious and conscientious objectors. If we believe that the existing standards for determining death reflect the facts about organ donors being dead, it seems as if the law is accommodating views that are false for strange reasons.

If we accommodate different views about death but the law claims only that the determination of death in the case of vital organ transplantation is a legal fiction, then there is coherence in the law. The determination of death is set by virtue of a policy choice, but it does not mean that someone with "total brain failure" is actually dead.

In other words, the application of the law does not require that the truth of death is established and universally endorsed, but that certain circumstances be treated as sufficient to determine the eligibility of patients for vital organ donation. The law about the determination of death would not establish or even have to consider the (scientific) truth about death. Under this approach, then, those who insist that vital organ donors must be dead in fact as well as legally dead are free to understand individuals diagnosed as "brain dead" as actually being dead under some definition of death. Others who regard these individuals as biologically alive will justify procuring vital organs from these donors on the grounds that they are legally dead and no harm or wrong is done to them when they or their authorized surrogates have decided to donate their organs. Still others might decide that these individuals are alive and that organs should not be taken from them, and will refuse to consent to organ donation for themselves or their families on that basis. Similarly, with the practice of DCDD, some can interpret these donors as dead in fact as well as legally dead when death is declared a few minutes after their hearts have stopped beating. Others can take the stance that we do not know that they are dead at this point but that they can be considered legally dead; therefore it is legitimate to procure organs on the grounds that no harm or wrong is done to these individuals, given valid decisions to stop life-sustaining treatment and donate organs.

Such a pluralistic approach to the status quo will not satisfy everyone. Some will believe that "brain-dead" individuals are not in fact dead and that therefore they should not be used as organ donors because doing so is wrongfully killing them. They remain free to choose not to become organ donors themselves should they become "brain dead" and not to authorize organ transplantation for family members who have not chosen to donate in the event of a diagnosis of brain death. Yet they may still be morally opposed to the legal practice of vital organ transplantation from "brain-dead" donors. They are essentially in the same position as those who decry the legal practice of abortion as murder. In any case, all can recognize the law as a common normative standard for governing society, even when the law permits practices that some regard as immoral. In sum, the legal fictions approach to vital organ transplantation contributes to pluralistic understandings of our current practices, notwithstanding the fact that ethical disagreement over these practices is likely to continue.

REVISITING THE DEAD DONOR RULE

Kierkegaard famously declared that life is lived forward but understood backward. This is true not only of biography but also of human history, including the history of medical ethics. Like any insightful aphorism, this one can't be taken literally. It is not the case that we have no understanding of what we are doing in the present as we move toward the future; however, our present understanding is subject to revision as we look back. The retrospective examination can produce the judgment that we were operating under a misconception. Such is our judgment about the history of medical ethics relating to organ transplantation. Medical ethics, so to speak, took the wrong turn in attempting to legitimize organ donation by revising or updating the standards for determining death. Instead of addressing the question of when it is ethical to procure vital organs, the question was begged by presuming the necessity of the DDR—a corollary of the traditional norm that doctors must not kill. Given this presumption, the path of least resistance was to change the standards for determining death in a way that permitted vital organ donation. It is probable that some of the key actors in this history of medical ethics, such as Henry Beecher, understood, at least dimly, that this is what they were doing. In any case, this way of dealing with the ethical challenges posed by the new technologies of intensive care medicine and organ transplantation was facilitated by the presumed view that the determination of death lies within the province of medical expertise. Hence, searching ethical inquiry was obviated by technical reconstruction of medical standards for determining death. This process included the diagnosis of "brain death" and declaring the propriety of pronouncing death on the basis of circulatory criteria only a short interval after asystole.

We live with this legacy of linking vital organ donation to the definition of, and standards for determining, death. From a theoretical perspective it would be desirable to break the link because, in fact, current practices are procuring organs from still-living patient-donors. Practically, however, this is difficult to achieve. For this reason we have recommended a legal fictions approach as a halfway house in the evolution of medical ethics and the law. We see this as a temporary expedient in the process of reconstructing medical ethics at the end of life. It is halfway to abandoning the dead donor rule. As we have argued, it is also a pragmatic compromise that accommodates the pluralism of current ethical views about when it is appropriate to procure vital organs.

What, then, is the status of the DDR within the legal fictions approach? We understand the DDR as strictly a legal rule, with no inherent ethical significance. Vital organs can be procured from those who are legally dead—a status that does not, in fact, coincide with death from either the perspectives of common sense or biomedicine. This approach is not arbitrary in light of the sound ethical justification under specified conditions for procuring vital organs from patient-donors who are still living, which we developed in Chapter 6. This justification applies to our current practices of organ transplantation. We see the legal fictions approach as progressive because, as a step in the evolution to greater transparency, it weakens the link between the ethics of organ transplantation and standards for determining death. The dead donor rule is preserved but lacks moral force. As the legal fictions underlying our current practices become more widely acknowledged by professionals and the public, the "scaffolding" of the DDR, which is maintained only by virtue of legal fictions relating to the determination of death, may be seen as no longer practically necessary. And this could lead to the legal changes necessary to bring the law into harmony with a reconstructed medical ethics without appeal to fictions.

Epilogue

At the end of the book we return to where we began. Developments in medical technology in the mid-twentieth century posed exciting opportunities and perplexing challenges. We have focused here on the ethical implications of two related technological developments: life-sustaining treatment, epitomized by intensive care units, and organ transplantation. It is the fate of modern medicine that the use of life-saving technology goes hand in hand with physicians causing the death of patients, though this has not been acknowledged. The use of medical technology in the intensive care setting is accompanied by the need to make decisions to withdraw life support, thus causing the patient's death. Transplantation of vital organs, though nominally governed by the dead donor rule, has in fact involved organ procurement from still-living patients, thus also making this practice responsible for causing death. However, established medical ethics has not faced up to the truth and developed an honest ethical rationale for these practices.

It was, nevertheless, natural for clinicians and ethicists to face the ethical challenges of these new technologies in a conservative way, holding fast to the traditional norm that doctors must not kill and endorsing the dead donor rule. The power to sustain life in the face of systemic organ failure was accompanied by the need to decide when to stop life support. Initial concern with doctors causing the death of patients by stopping life-sustaining medical treatment was allayed by seeing this practice as merely allowing patients to die from their underlying disease or injury, thus preserving the prohibition on killing. The opportunity for organ transplantation, with the potential for long-term survival in the face of previously terminal disease, also put pressure on traditional medical ethics. Permitting vital organ donation was seen to require that the donor be dead; otherwise physicians would be responsible for killing some patients to save the lives of others. Patients on life support in an irreversible coma and unable to breathe on their own were seen as ideal candidates for transplanting vital organs, despite displaying the appearance of vitality.

Although promulgating a new conception of death diagnosed by neurological criteria was a radical innovation, it was easier to make what was perceived as a technical change in the determination of death than to modify the norm that doctors must not kill. The new conception of death emerged at the dawn of bioethics, when public deference to medical expertise remained in force.

The conservative preservation of traditional medical ethics in the face of these technological challenges served medicine and the public reasonably well. But this ethical consensus is based on a fragile intellectual foundation that has eroded in response to critical scrutiny. Many have thought that it is arbitrary to permit the withdrawal of life support but prohibit physician-assisted death by prescribing or administering lethal medication. In recent years assisted suicide and active euthanasia have been legalized in various jurisdictions. More pervasive erosion has occurred in the rationale for the determination of death by use of neurological criteria. Evidence has accumulated that those diagnosed as "brain dead" retain some brain functioning and, more significantly, they retain extensive functioning of the organism as a whole, in the form of circulation, respiration, metabolism, wound healing, fighting infection, and gestating a fetus—organismic functions that in point of fact do not require integration by the brain. Medicine relies on a biological conception of life and death, and within that framework no credible rationale has emerged for why "brain dead" bodies are dead. The practice of donation after circulatory determination of death (DCDD) also has strained credibility concerning adherence to the dead donor rule, insofar as it is impossible to be certain that circulation has irreversibly ceased within a few minutes after asystole.

In this book we have argued essentially that the "center cannot not hold" with respect to medical ethics at the end of life. There is no credible way to support the current practices of withdrawing life support and vital organ transplantation consistent with the traditional norm that doctors must never intentionally cause the death of patients and consistent with the dead donor rule. Modifying traditional medical ethics will not come easily, but there is no intellectually respectable alternative. We have no ability to predict the future, but it is hard to imagine that the ethical status quo can remain in force in the long run. Our critique of traditional medical ethics at the end of life is apt to be controversial and seem radical. We have argued that it is ethically legitimate for doctors to intervene in ways that cause the death of patients: by withdrawing life support for the sake of avoiding harm to them and respecting their preferences, and by procuring vital organs from still-living donors to save the lives of others under specified conditions. Legitimate practices of withdrawing treatment and vital organ transplantation hitherto have been justified by an appeal to morally biased judgments relating to causation and by fictions and fudges concerning the determination of death. However, they can, and should, be justified in an honest and straightforward way. But this requires abandoning the absolute norm that doctors must not kill and its corollary, the dead donor rule.

To a large extent the ethical approach that we have advanced here is conservative in practice. It does, however, open up ethical space for improving the outcomes of vital organ transplantation without harm or wrong to donors (by routinely procuring vital organs before withdrawing life support with valid consent) and, with due caution, instituting the practice of physician-assisted death, provided that adequate safeguards can be implemented. This is not the "brave new world" of medicine at the end of life; rather, it is the world we currently occupy, but seen through a different ethical lens, recognizing that adherence to traditional medical ethics is incoherent.

REFERENCES

Ad Hoc Committee of the Harvard Medical School to Examine the Definition of Brain Death. 1968. A definition of irreversible coma. *Journal of the American Medical Association* 205: 337–340.

Alicke, M. D. 1992. Culpable causation. *Journal of Personality and Social Psychology* 63: 368–378.

Arras, J. D. 1998. Physician-assisted suicide: A tragic choice. In: M. P. Battin, R. Rhodes, and A. Silvers, Eds., *Physician Assisted Suicide: Expanding the Debate*. New York: Routledge: 279–300.

Arras, J. D. 2001. A method in search of a purpose: The internal morality of medicine. *Journal of Medicine and Philosophy* 26: 643–662.

Baier, A. C. 1994. *Moral Prejudice*. Cambridge: Harvard University Press.

Barnard, C. N. 1967. The operation: A human cardiac transplant: An interim report of a successful operation performed at Groote Schuur Hospital, Cape Town. *South African Medical Journal* 41: 1271–1274.

Barnard, C. N. 1987. Reflections on the first heart transplant. *South African Medical Journal* 72 (December 5): 19.

Bartlett, R. H. 2009. ECMO Conference. Keystone, Colorado, February 2009.

Beauchamp, T. L. 1999. The failure of theories of personhood. *Kennedy Institute of Ethics Journal* 9: 309–324.

Beauchamp, T. L., and J. F. Childress. 2009. *Principles of Biomedical Ethics*, 6th ed. New York: Oxford University Press.

Bentham, J. 1838/1977. *Preface for the Second Edition* to *A Comment on the Commentaries and a Fragment of Government* (J.H. Burns and H.L.A. Hart, eds. Oxford: Oxford University Press, 1977, first published in 1838), 509.

Beresford, H. R. 1999. Brain death. *Neurology Clinics* 17(2): 295.

Bergelson, V. 2010. Consent to Harm. In: F. G. Miller and A. Wertheimer, Eds., *The Ethics of Consent: Theory and Practice*. New York: Oxford University Press: 163–192.

Bernat, J. L. 1992. How much of the brain must die in brain death? *Journal of Clinical Ethics* 3: 21–26.

Bernat, J. L. 1998. A defense of the whole-brain concept of death. *Hastings Center Report* 28(2): 14–23.

Bernat, J. L. 2006a. The whole-brain concept of death remains optimum public policy. *Journal of Law, Medicine & Ethics* 34(1): 35–43.

Bernat, J. L. 2006b. Are organ donors after cardiac death really dead? *Journal of Clinical Ethics* 17(2): 122–132.

Bernat, J. L. 2006c. Chronic disorder of consciousness. *Lancet* 367: 1181–1192.

Bernat, J. L. 2010a. Are donors after circulatory death really dead and does it matter? Yes and Yes. *Chest* 138: 13–16.

Bernat, J. L. 2010b. How the distinction between "irreversible" and "permanent" illuminates circulatory-respiratory death determination. *Journal of Medicine and Philosophy* 35(June): 242–255.

Bernat, J. L., C. M. Culver, and B. Gert. 1981. On the definition and criterion of death. *Annals of Internal Medicine* 94: 389–394.

Bernat, J. L., A. M. D'Alessandro, F. K. Port, et al. 2006. Report of a National Conference on Donation after cardiac death. *American Journal of Transplantation* 6(2): 281–291.

Bernat, J. L., A. M. Capron, T. P. Bleck, et al. 2010. The circulatory-respiratory determination of death in organ donation. *Critical Care Medicine* 38(3): 963–970.

Bernstein, R. J. 2010. *The Pragmatic Turn*. Cambridge, U.K.: Polity Press.

Betzold, M. 1993. *Appointment with Doctor Death*. Troy, MI: Momentum Books.

Bickenbach, J. E. 1998. Disability and life-ending decisions. In: M. P. Battin, R. Rhodes, and A. Silvers, Eds., *Physician Assisted Suicide: Expanding the Debate*. New York: Routledge: 123–132.

Bix, B. H. 2009. Law and language: How words mislead us. Reappointment Lecture to the Frederick W. Thomas Chair, University of Minnesota (April 7, 2009), available at http://ssrn.com/abstract=1376366.

Bosshard, G., et al. 2006. Intentionally hastening death by withholding or withdrawing treatment. *Wiener Klinische Wochenschrift* 118: 322–326.

Boucek, M. M., C. Mashburn, S. M. Dunn, et al. 2008. Pediatric heart transplantation after declaration of cardiocirculatory death. *New England Journal of Medicine* 359(7): 709–714.

Brilli, R. J., and D. Bigos. 2000. Apnea threshold and pediatric brain death. *Critical Care Medicine* 28: 1257.

Brock, D. W. 1992. Voluntary active euthanasia. *Hastings Center Report* 22(2): 10–22.

Brock, D. W. 1993. *Life and Death*. Cambridge, U.K.: Cambridge University Press.

Brock, D. W. 1999. The role of the public in public policy on the definition of death. In: S. J. Youngner, R. M. Arnold, and R. Schapiro, Eds., *The Definition of Death*. Baltimore: The Johns Hopkins Press: 293–307.

Brody, B. 1996. Withdrawal of treatment versus killing of patients. In: T. L. Beauchamp, Ed., *Intending Death: The Ethics of Assisted Suicide and Euthanasia*. Upper Saddle River, NJ: Prentice Hall: 90–103.

Brody, H. 1981. *Ethical Dimensions in Medicine*. Boston: Little, Brown.

Brubaker, R. 2005. Taking exception to the new corporate discharge exceptions. 13 *American Bankrupcy Institute Law Review* 757.

Bryne, P.A., S. Oreilly, et al. 1979. Brain death—an opposing viewpoint. *Journal of the American Medical Association* 242: 1985–1990.

Callahan, D. 1992. When self-determination runs amok. *Hastings Center Report* 22(2): 52–55.

Callahan, D. 1993. *The Troubled Dream of Life*. New York: Simon & Schuster.

Callahan, D. 1996. The goals of medicine: Setting new priorities. *Hastings Center Report* 25(6): S1–S26.

Capron, A. M. 1999. The bifurcated legal standard for determining death: Does it work? In: S. J. Youngner, R. M. Arnold, and R. Schapiro, Eds., *The Definition of Death*. Baltimore: The Johns Hopkins Press: 117–136.

Capron, A. M. 2001. Brain death—well settled yet still unresolved. *New England Journal of Medicine* 344: 1244–1246.

Charo, A R. 1999. Dusk, dawn, and defining death: Legal classifications and biological categories. In: S. J. Youngner, R. M. Arnold, and R. Schapiro, Eds., *The Definition of Death*. Baltimore: The Johns Hopkins Press: 277–292.

Chervenak, F. A., and L. B. McCullough. 2006. Why the Groningen Protocol should be rejected. *Hastings Center Report* 36(5): 30–33.

CNN Wire Staff. 2010. Lou Gehrig's victim: Kill me for my organs. www.cnn/2010/HEALTH/07/29/georgia.right.to.die/index.html?hpt=Sbin, accessed 7/30/09.

Collaborative Study. 1977. An appraisal of the criteria of cerebral death, a summary statement: A collaborative study. *Journal of the American Medical Association* 237: 982–986.

Collins, T., and L. Leff. 2009. Wounded Oakland officer brain-dead. *The Washington Post*, March 23, 2009: A4.

Combs v. Int'l Ins. Co. 2004. 354 F. 3d 568, 599 (6th Cir. Ky.).

Dagi, T. F. 1992. Commentary on "How much of the brain must dies in brain death?" *Journal of Clinical Ethics* 3: 27–28.

Dalgleish, D. 2000. Brain stem death: Healthcare workers have difficulty accepting current management. *British Medical Journal* 321: 635.

Damasio, A. 2010. *Self Comes to Mind*. New York: Pantheon Books.

de Groot, Y. J., and E. J. Kompanje. 2010. Dead donor rule and organ procurement. *Pediatric Critical Care Medicine* 11(2): 314–315.

DeVita, M. A. 2001. The death watch: Certifying death using cardiac criteria. *Progress in Transplantation* 11(1): 58–66.

DeVita, M. A., and J. V. Snyder. 1993. Development of the University of Pittsburgh Medical Center Policy for the care of terminally ill patients who may become organ donors after death following the removal of life support. *Kennedy Institute of Ethics Journal* 3: 131–143.

DeVita, M. A., J. V. Snyder, R. M. Arnold, and L. A. Siminoff. 2000. Observations of withdrawal of life-sustaining treatment from patients who became non-heart-beating organ donors. *Critical Care Medicine* 28(6): 1709–1712.

Diflo, T. 2004. Use of organs from executed Chinese prisoners. *Lancet* 364: 30–31.

Dosemeci, L., M Cengiz, et al. 2004. Frequency of spinal reflex movements in brain dead patients. *Transplantation Proceedings* 36(1): 17–19.

Douglas, C., I. Kerridge, and R. Ankeny. 2008. Managing intentions: The end-of-life administration of analgesics and sedatives, and the possibility of slow euthanasia. *Bioethics* 22: 388–396.

Dubois, J. M., and T. Schmidt 2003. Does the public support organ donation using higher brain-death criteria? *Journal of Clinical Ethics* 14(1–2): 26.

Dumit, J. 2004. *Picturing Personhood: Brain Scans and Biomedical Identity*. Princeton: Princeton University Press.

Dworkin, G. 2002. Patients and prisoners: The ethics of lethal injection. *Analysis* 62: 181–189.

Dworkin, R. 1993. *Life's Dominion*. New York: Alfred A. Knopf.

Dworkin, R. 2010. NYRblog, "The Devastating Decision," available at http://blogs.nybooks.com/post/354384835/the-devastating-decision.

Eddy, D. M. 1994. A piece of my mind. A conversation with my mother. *Journal of the American Medical Association* 272: 179–181.

Emanuel, E. J. 1999. What is the great benefit of legalizing euthanasia or physician-assisted suicide? *Ethics* 109: 629–642.

Engelhardt, H. T. 1975. Defining death: A philosophical problem for medicine and law. *American Review of Respiratory Disease* 112: 587–590.

Englehardt, H. T. 1986. *The Foundations of Bioethics*. New York: Oxford University Press.

Fabre, C. 2006. *Whose Body Is It Anyway?* Oxford: Oxford University Press.

Fackler, J. C., and R. D. Truog. 1987. Is brain death really cessation of all intracranial function? *Journal Pediatrics* 110: 84–86.

Faden, R. R., and T. L. Beauchamp. 1986. *A History and Theory of Informed Consent*. New York: Oxford University Press.

Feinberg, J. 1984. *Harm to Others*. New York: Oxford University Press.

Feinberg, J. 1986. *Harm to Self*. New York: Oxford University Press.

Feldman, F. 1992. *Confrontations with the Reaper: A Philosophical Study of the Nature and Value of Death*. New York: Oxford University Press.

Festinger, L., and J. M. Carlsmith. 1959. Cognitive consequences of forced compliance. *Journal of Abnormal and Social Psychology* 58: 203–211.

Foot, P. 1994. Killing and allowing to die. In: B. Steinbock and A. Norcross, Eds., *Killing and Letting Die*, 2nd ed. New York: Fordham University Press: 280–289.

Frank, J. 1973. *Courts on Trial: Myth and Reality in American Justice*. Princeton: Princeton University Press: 147.

Friedlander, H. 1995. *The Origins of Nazi Genocide: From Euthanasia to the Final Solution*. Chapel Hill: University of North Carolina Press.

Fuller, L. 1967. *Legal Fictions*. Stanford, CA: Stanford University Press.

Gay, P. 1988. *Freud*. New York: Norton.

Gaylin, W., L. R. Kass, E. D. Pellegrino, and M. Siegler. 1988. Doctors must not kill. *Journal of the American Medical Association* 259: 2139–2140.

Gert, B., J. L. Bernat, and R. P. Mogielnicki. 1994. Distinguishing between patients' refusals and requests. *Hastings Center Report* 24(4): 13–15.

Gervais, K. G. 1986. *Redefining Death*. New Haven: Yale University Press.

Glannon, W. 2007. *Bioethics and the Brain*. New York: Oxford University Press.

Gravel, M. T., J. D. Arenas, R. Chenault, 2nd, et al. 2004. Kidney transplantation from organ donors following cardiopulmonary death using extracorporeal membrane oxygenation support. *Annals of Transplantation* 9(1): 57–58.

Green, M. B. and D. Wikler. 1980. Brain death and personal identity. *Philosophy and Public Affairs* 9: 105–133.

Greenberg, G. 2001. As good as dead. *New Yorker*. August 13, 2001.

Greene, J. 2009. Fruit flies of the moral mind. In: M. Brockman, Ed., *What's Next? Dispatches on the Future of Science*. New York: Vintage Books. 104–115.

Guidelines for the Determination of Death. 1981. Report of the medical consultants on the diagnosis of death to the President's Commission for the Study of Ethical Problems in Medicine and Biomedical and Behavioral Research. *Journal of the American Medical Association* 246: 2184–2186.

Halevy, A., and B. Brody. 1993. Brain death: Reconciling definitions, criteria, and tests. *Annals of Internal Medicine* 119: 519–525.

Hall, M., F. F. Trachtenberg, and E. Dugan. 2005. The impact of patient trust on legalizing physician aid in dying. *Journal of Medical Ethics* 31: 693–697.

Harmon, L. 1990. Falling off the vine: Legal fictions and the doctrine of substituted judgment. 100 *Yale Law Journal* 1.

Hart, H. L. A., and T. Honore. 1985. *Causation in the Law*, 2nd ed. New York: Oxford University Press.

Hershenov, D. B., and J. J. Delaney.. 2009. Mandatory autopsies and organ conscription. *Kennedy Institute of Ethics Journal* 19: 367–391.

Hornby, K., L. Hornby, and S. D. Shemie. 2010. A systematic review of autoresuscitation after cardiac arrest. *Critical Care Medicine* 38(5): 1246–1253.

Huxtable, R., and M. Moller. 2007. "Setting a principled boundary"? Euthanasia as a response to "life fatigue." *Bioethics* 21: 117–126.

Institute of Medicine. 2000. *Non-Heart-Beating Organ Transplantation: Practice and Protocols*. Washington, D.C.: National Academy Press.

Jonas, H. 1970. Philosophical reflections on experimenting with human subjects. In: Freund PA, ed. *Experimentation with Human Subjects* . New York: George Braziller: 1–31.

Jonas, H. 1974. Against the stream: Comments on the definition and redefinition of death. In: H. Jonas. *Philosophical Essays*. Chicago: University of Chicago Press: 132–140.

Jonsen, A. R. 1989. Ethical issues in organ transplantation. In: R. M. Veatch, Ed., *Medical Ethics*. Boston: Jones and Bartlett: 229–252.

Kamm, F. M. 1996. *Morality, Mortality*, Volume II. New York: Oxford University Press.

Kass, L. R. 1985. *Toward a More Natural Science*. New York: Free Press.

Kass, L. R. 1989. Neither for love nor money: Why doctors must not kill. *The Public Interest* 94: 25–46.

Kato, T., A. Tokumaru, et al. 1991. Assessment of brain death in children by means of P-31 MR spectroscopy: Preliminary note. Work in progress [see comments]. *Radiology* 179: 95–99.

Keep, P. J. 2000. Anaesthesia for organ donation in the brainstem dead. *Anaesthesia* 55(6): 590.

Khushf, G. 2010. A matter of respect: A defense of the dead donor rule and of "whole-brain" criterion for determination of death. *Journal of Medicine and Philosophy* 35: 330–364.

King, L. 2005. CNN LARRY KING LIVE: Interview with Jason, Justin Torres.

Kleinig, J. 2010. The nature of Consent. In: F. G. Miller and A. Wertheimer, *The Ethics of Consent: Theory and Practice*. New York: Oxford University Press: 3–24.

Korein, J. 1978. The problem of brain death: Development and history. *Annals of the New York Academy of Sciences* 315: 19–38.

Kunin, J. 2004. Brain death: Revisiting rabbinic opinions in light of current knowledge. *Tradition* 38(4): 48–62.

Lagnado, D. A., and S. Channon 2008. Judgments of cause and blame: The effects of intentionality and foreseeability. *Cognition* 108: 754–770.

Lane, A., A. Westbrook, et al. 2004. Maternal brain death: Medical, ethical and legal issues. Intensive Care Medicine 30(3–4): 1484–1486.

Larkin, P. 1977. Aubade. In: A. Thwaite, Ed., *Philip Larkin. Collected Poems*. New York: Farrar Strauss Giroux, 1988: 208.

Lindemann, H., and M. Verkerk. 2008. Ending the life of a newborn: The Groningen Protocol. *Hastings Center Report* 38(1): 42–51.

Lizza, J. P. 2006. *Persons, Humanity, and the Definition of Death*. Baltimore: Johns Hopkins University Press.

Lizza, J. P. 2009a. And she's not only merely dead, she's really most sincerely dead. *Hastings Center Report* 39(5): 5–6.

Lizza, J. P. 2009b. Commentary on "The incoherence of determining death by neurological criteria." *Kennedy Institute of Ethics Journal* 19: 393–395.

Machado, C., and Korein, J. 2009. Irreversibility: Cardiac death versus brain death. *Reviews in the Neurosciences* 20(3–4): 199–292.

Macklem, P. T., and A. Seely. 2010. Towards a definition of life. *Perspectives in Biology and Medicine* 53: 330–340.

Magliocca, J. F., J. C. Magee, S. A. Rowe, et al. 2005. Extracorporeal support for organ donation after cardiac death effectively expands the donor pool. *Journal of Trauma* 58(6): 1095–1101; discussion 1101–1102.

Marcus, R. 2010. The high court's shoddy scholarship. *Washington Post*, January 23, 2010, at A13.

Marquis, D. 2010. Are DCD donors dead? *Hastings Center Report* 40(3): 24–31.

Matta, B. 2000. The implications of anaesthetising the brainstem dead: 2--Reply. *Anaesthesia* 55(7): 695–696.

McIntyre, A. 2009. Doctrine of Double Effect. *Stanford Encyclopedia of Philosophy*. http://plato.stanford.edu/entries/double-effect/, accessed 11/4/09.

McMahan, J. 2002. *The Ethics of Killing*. New York: Oxford University Press.

Medical Royal Colleges and Their Faculties in the United Kingdom. 1976. Diagnosis of brain death. Statement issued by the honorary secretary of the Conference of Medical Royal Colleges and Their Faculties in the United Kingdom on 11 October 1976. *British Medical Journal* 2: 1187–1188.

Merker B. 2007. Consciousness without a cerebral cortex: A challenge for neuroscience and medicine. *Behavioral and Brain Sciences* 30: 63–81.

Mill, J. S. 1859. On liberty. In: J. S. Mill, *Utilitarianism, Liberty and Representative Government*. Everyman Library. London: J.M. Dent, 1971.

Miller, F. G. 1991. Is active killing of patients always wrong? *Journal of Clinical Ethics* 2: 130–132.

Miller, F. G. 2009a. A planned death in the family. *Hastings Center Report* 39(2): 28–30.

Miller, F. G. 2009b. Death and organ donation: Back to the future. *Journal of Medical Ethics* 35: 616–620.

Miller, F. G., and H. Brody. 1995. Professional integrity and physician-assisted death. *Hastings Center Report* 25(3): 8–17.

Miller, F. G, and H. Brody. 2001. The internal morality of medicine: An evolutionary perspective. *Journal of Medicine and Philosophy* 26: 581–599.

Miller, F. G., and H. Brody. 2003. A critique of clinical equipoise: Therapeutic misconception in the ethics of clinical trials. *Hastings Center Report* 33(3): 19–28.

Miller, F. G., and D. L. Rosenstein. 2003. The therapeutic orientation to clinical trials. *New England Journal of Medicine* 348: 1383–1386.

Miller, F. G., and A. Wertheimer. 2010. Preface to a theory of consent transactions: Beyond valid consent. In: F. G. Miller and A. Wertheimer. Eds., *The Ethics of Consent: Theory and Practice*. New York: Oxford University Press: 79–105.

Miller, F. G., et al. 1994. Regulating physician-assisted death. *New England Journal of Medicine* 331: 119–123.

Miller, F. G., and Truog, R. D. 2008. Rethinking the ethics of vital organ donations. *Hastings Center Report* 38(6): 38–46.

Miller, F. G., and Truog, R. D. 2009. The incoherence of determining death by neurological criteria: Commentary on *Controversies in the Determination of Death*, A White Paper by the President's Council on Bioethics. *Kennedy Institutes of Ethics Journal* 19: 185–93.

Miller, F. G., and Truog, R. D. 2010. Decapitation and the definition of death. *Journal of Medical Ethics* 36: 632–634.

Miller, F. G., Truog, R. D., and Brock, D. W. 2010a. Moral fictions and medical ethics. *Bioethics* 24: 453–460.

Miller, F. G., Truog, R. D., and Brock, D. W. 2010b. The dead donor rule: can it withstand critical scrutiny? *Journal of Medicine and Philosophy* 35: 299–312.

Molinari, G. F., U. S. Department of Health, et al. 1980. The NINCDS Collaborative Study of Brain Death: A historical perspective. *NINCDS Monograph No. 24. NIH publication No. 81–2286*: 1–32.

Mollaret, P., and M. Goulon. 1959. Le coma depasse. *Revue Neurologie* 101: 3–15.

Monti, M. M., M. R. Coleman, and A. M. Owen. 2009. Neuroimaging and the vegetative state: Resolving the behavioral assessment dilemma? *Annals of the New York Academy of Sciences* 1157: 81–89.

Monti, M. M., A. Vanhaudenhuyse, et al. 2010. Willful modulation of brain activity in disorders of consciousness. *New England Journal of Medicine* 362: 579–589.

Morray, J. P., E. J. Krane, et al. 1987. Brain death? *Pediatrics* 79: 1057.

Munsell, M. G. 1997. The declaratory judgment act's actual controversy requirement: Should a patent owner's promise not to sue deprive the court of jurisdiction? *Super Sack Manufacturing Corp. v. Chase Packaging Corp.* 1, 62 Mo. *Law Review* 573: 580–582.

Nachev, P., and P. M. S. Hacker. 2010. Covert cognition in the persistent vegetative state. *Progress in Neurobiology* 91: 68–76.

Nelson, J. 2009. Dealing death and retrieving organs. *Journal of Bioethical Inquiry* 6: 285–291.

Noe, A. 2009. *Out of Our Heads*. New York: Hill and Wang.

Okie S. 2005. Physician-assisted suicide—Oregon and beyond. *New England Journal of Medicine* 352: 1627–1630.

Olick, R. S. 1991. Brain death, religious freedom, and public policy: New Jersey's landmark legislative initiative. *Kennedy Institute of Ethics Journal* 1: 275–288.

Olick, R. S., Braun, E. A., and J. Potash. 2009. Accommodating religious and moral objections to neurological death. *Journal of Clinical Ethics* 20(2): 183–191.

Outka, G. 2002. The ethics of human cell research. *Kennedy Institute of Ethics Journal* 12: 175–213.

Owen, A. M., M. R. Coleman, M. Boly, et al. 2006. Detecting awareness in the vegetative state. *Science* 313: 1402.

Panksepp, J., T. Fuchs, V. A. Garcia, and A. Lesiak. 2007. Does any aspect of mind survive brain damage that typically leads to a persistent vegetative state? Ethical considerations. *Philosophy, Ethics, and Humanities in Medicine* 2: 32.

Patterson, D. R., et al. 1993. When life support is questioned early in the care of patients with cervical-level quadriplegia. *New England Journal of Medicine* 328: 506–509.

Pence, G. E. 1995. *Classic Cases in Medical Ethics*, 2nd ed. New York: McGraw-Hill: 3–33.

Pernick, M. S. 1988. Back from the grave: Recurring controversies over defining and diagnosing death in history. In: R. M. Zaner. Ed., *Death: Beyond Whole-Brain Criteria*. Boston: Kluwer Academic Publishers: 17–74.

Plum, F., and J. B. Posner. 2007. *The Diagnosis of Stupor and Coma*, 4th ed. New York: Oxford University Press.

Pope Pius XII. 1957a. The prolongation of life. The Pope Speaks: 393, 396.

Pope Pius XII. 1957b. Address to an international congress of anesthesiologists. http:// www.lifeissues.net/writers/doc/doc_31resuscitation.html. Accessed 11/5/09.

Poulton, B., and M. Garfield. 2000. The implications of anaesthetising the brainstem dead: 1. *Anaesthesia* 55(7): 695.

Powner, D. J., and I. M. Bernstein. 2003. Extended somatic support for pregnant women after brain death. *Critical Care Medicine* 31: 1241–1249.

President's Commission for the Study of Ethical Problems in Biomedical Medicine and Biomedical and Behavioral Research. 1981. *Defining Death: A Report on the Medical, Legal, and Ethical Issues in the Determination of Death* . Washington, DC: Government Printing Office.

President's Commission for the Study of Ethical Problems in Medicine and Biomedical and Behavioral Research. 1983. *Deciding to Forego Life-Sustaining Treatment*. Washington, D.C.: Government Printing Office.

President's Council on Bioethics. 2008. *Controversies in the Determination of Death*. Washington, D.C. www.bioethics.gov.

Proctor, R. N. 1988. *Racial Hygiene: Medicine under the Nazis*. Cambridge, MA: Harvard University Press.

Que, C. L., C. M. Kenyon R. Olivenstein, et al. 2001. Homeokinesis and short-term variability of human airway caliber. *Journal of Applied Physiology* 91: 1131–1141.

Quill, T. E. 1993. The ambiguity of clinical intentions. *New England Journal of Medicine* 329: 1039–1040.

Quill, T. E., et al. 2009. Last-resort options for palliative sedation. *Annals of Internal Medicine* 151: 421–424.

Ravitsky V. 2005. Timers on ventilators. *BMJ* 330: 415–417.

Reiser, S. J. 1993. Science, pedagogy, and the transformation of empathy in medicine. In: H. M. Spiro et al., Eds., *Empathy and the Practice of Medicine*. New Haven: Yale University Press: 121–134.

Repertinger, S., W. P. Fitzgibbons, et al. 2006. Long survival following bacterial meningitis-associated brain destruction. *Journal of Child Neurology* 21(7): 591–595.

Rich, B. A. 1997. Postmodern personhood: A matter of consciousness. *Bioethics* 11: 206–216.

Rietjens, J. A. C., et al. 2007. Using drugs to end life without an explicit request of the patient. *Death Studies* 31: 205–221.

Rietjens, J. A. C., et al. 2009. Two decades of research on euthanasia from the Netherlands: What have we learnt and what questions remain? *Bioethical Inquiry* 6: 271–283.

Robertson, J. 1999. The dead donor rule. *Hastings Center Report* 29(6): 6–14.

Rodin, E., S. Tahir, et al. 1985. Brainstem death. *Clinical Electroencephalography* 16: 63–71.

Rosen, J. Roberts versus Roberts. *New Republic*, March 11, 2010: 17.

Rosner, F. 1999. The definition of death in Jewish law. In: S. J. Youngner, R.M. Arnold, and R. Schapiro. Eds., *The Definition of Death*. Baltimore: John Hopkins University Press: 210–221.

Sanchez-Fructuouso, A. L., et al. 2006. Victims of cardiac arrest occurring outside the hospital: A source of transplantable kidneys. *Annals of Internal Medicine* 145: 157–164.

Sanghavi, D. 2009. When does death start? *New York Times Magazine*, December 20, 2009.

Sass, H. M. 1992. Criteria for death: Self-determination and public policy. *Journal of Medicine and Philosophy* 17: 445–454.

Schmidt, T. C. 2004. The Ohio study in light of national data and clinical experience. *Kennedy Institute of Ethics Journal* 14: 235–240.

Segev, D. L., A. D. Muzaale, B. S. Caffo, et al. 2010. Perioperative mortality and long-term survival following live kidney donation. *Journal of the American Medical Association* 303: 959–966.

Shah S. K., and F. G. Miller. 2010. Can we handle the truth? Legal fictions in the determination of death. *American Journal of Law & Medicine* 36: 540–585.

Shewmon, D. A. 1987. The probability of inevitability: The inherent impossibility of validating criteria for brain death or "irreversibility" through clinical studies. *Statistics in Medicine* 6: 535–553.

Shewmon, D.A. 1997. Recovery from "brain death": A neurologist's apologia. *Linacre Quarterly* 64(1): 30–96.

Shewmon, D. A. 1998. Chronic "brain death"—Meta-analysis and conceptual consequences. *Neurology* 51(6): 1538–1545.

Shewmon, D. A. 1999. Spinal shock and brain death: Somatic pathophysiological equivalence and implications for the integrative-unity rationale. *Spinal Cord* 37(5): 313–324.

Shewmon, D. A. 2001. The brain and somatic integration: Insights into the standard biological rationale for equating "brain death" with death. *Journal of Medicine and Philosophy* 26: 457–478.

Shewmon, D. A. 2004. The "critical organ" for the organism as a whole: Lessons from the lowly spinal cord. *Advances in Experimental Medicine and Biology* 550: 23–41.

Shewmon, D. A. 2009. Brain death: Can it be resuscitated? *Hastings Center Report* 39(2): 18–23.

Shewmon, D. A., G. L. Holmes, and P. A. Byrne. 1999. Consciousness in congenitally decorticate children: Developmental vegetative state as self-fulfilling prophecy. *Developmental Medcine & Child Neurology* 41: 364–374.

Siminoff, L. A., C. Burant, and S. J.Youngner. 2004. Death and organ procurement: Public beliefs and attitudes. *Social Science & Medicine* 59: 2325–2334.

Singer, P. 1993. *Practice Ethics*, 2nd ed. New York: Cambridge University Press.

Singer, P. 2003. Voluntary euthanasia: A utilitarian perspective. *Bioethics* 17: 526–541.

Sprung, C. L., D. Ledoux, H. H. Bulow, et al. 2008. Relieving suffering or intentionally hastening death: Where do you draw the line? *Critical Care Medicine* 36: 8–13.

Stein, R. 2010. Project to get transplant organs from ER patients raises ethical questions. *New York Times* March 15, 2010: A1.

Steinberg, A ,and M. Hersch. 1995. Decapitation of a pregnant sheep: A contribution to the brain death controversy. *Transplantation Proceedings* 27: 1886–1887.

Steinbock, B., and A. Norcross. 1994. *Killing and Letting Die*, 2nd ed. New York: Fordham University Press.

Steinbrook, R. 2007. Organ donation after cardiac death. *New England Journal of Medicine* 357(3): 209–213.

Stevens, M. L. T. 2000. *Bioethics in America*. Baltimore: Johns Hopkins University Press.

Strung, C. L., et al. 2008. Relieving suffering or intentionally hastening death: Where do you draw the line? *Critical Care Medicine* 36: 8–13.

Supreme Court of New Jersey. 1976. In the matter of Karen Quinlan. In: B. Steinbock and A. Norcross, 1994. *Killing and Letting Die*, 2nd ed. New York: Fordham University Press: 51–78.

Tauber, A.I. 2009. *Science and the Quest for Meaning*. Waco, TX: Baylor University Press.

Tavris, C., and E. Aronson. 2007. *Mistakes Were Made: (But Not by Me)*. Orlando, FL: Harcourt, Brace: 13–20.

Truog, R. D. 1997. Is it time to abandon brain death? *Hastings Center Report* 27(1): 29–37.

Truog, R. D. 2007. Brain death—too flawed to endure, too ingrained to abandon. *Journal of Law, Medicine & Ethics* 35: 273–281.

Truog, R. D., and J. C. Fackler. 1992. Rethinking brain death. *Critical Care Medicine* 20: 1705–1713.

Truog, R. D., and W. M. Robinson. 2003. Role of brain death and the dead-donor rule in the ethics of organ transplantation. *Critical Care Medicine* 31: 2391–2396.

Truog, R. D. and F. G. Miller. 2008. The dead donor rule and organ donation. *New England Journal of Medicine* 359: 674–675.

Truog, R. D., and F. G. Miller. 2010. Counterpoint: Are donors after circulatory death really dead, and does it matter? No and not really. *Chest* 138: 16–18.

Truog, R. D., et al. 2001. Recommendations for end-of-life care in the intensive care unit: The ethics committee of the Society of Critical Care Medicine. *Critical Care Medicine* 29: 2332–2348.

Truog, R. D., M. L. Campbell, J. R. Curtis, et al. 2008. Recommendations for end-of-life care in the intensive care unit: A consensus by the American College of Critical Care Medicine. *Critical Care Medicine* 36: 953–963.

University of Pittsburgh Medical Center. 1993. Policy and Procedure Manual: Management of terminally ill patients who may become organ donors after death. *Kennedy Institute of Ethics Journal* 3: A1–A15.

UNOS. 2010. Available from http://unos.org/data/.

Vacco v. Quill. 1997. In: M. P. Battin, R. Rhodes, and A. Silvers, Eds., *1998. Physician Assisted Suicide: Expanding the Debate.* New York: Routledge.

van der Maas, P., and L. E. Emanuel. 1998. Factual findings. In: L. Emanuel, Ed., *Regulating How We Die.* Cambridge, MA: Harvard University Press: 151–174.

van der Maas, P. J., L. Pijnenborg, and J. J. van Delden. 1995. Changes in Dutch opinions on active euthanasia, 1966 through 1991. *Journal of the American Medical Association* 273: 1411–1414.

Vardis, R., and M. M. Pollack. 1998. Increased apnea threshold in a pediatric patient with suspected brain death. *Critical Care Medicine* 26: 1917–1919.

Veatch, R. M. 1975. The whole-brain oriented concept of death: An outmoded philosophical formulation. *Journal of Thanatology* 3: 13–30.

Veatch, R. M. 1992. Brain death and slippery slopes. *Journal of Clinical Ethics* 3: 181–187.

Veatch, R. M. 2008. Donating hearts after cardiac death—reversing the irreversible. *New England Journal of Medicine* 369: 672–673.

Veatch, R. M. 2010. Transplanting hearts after death measured by cardiac criteria: The challenge to the dead donor rule. *Journal of Medicine and Philosophy* 35(June): 313–329.

Velmans, M. 2009. *Understanding Consciousness*, 2nd ed. New York: Routledge.

Wang, M., and X. Wang. 2010. Organ donation by capital prisoners in China: Reflections on Confucian ethics. *Journal of Medicine and Philosophy* 35: 197–2010.

Wertheimer, A. 1996. *Exploitation.* Princeton, NJ: Princeton University Press.

Wijdicks, E. F. M. 2002. Brain death worldwide—accepted fact but no global consensus in diagnostic criteria. *Neurology* 58(1): 20–25.

Wijdicks, E. F., and E. A. Pfeifer. 2008. Neuropathology of brain death in the modern transplant era. *Neurology* 70: 1234–1237.

Wikler, D. I. 1984. Conceptual issues in the definition of death: A guide for public policy. *Theoretical Medicine* 5: 167–180.

Wikler, D., and A. J. Weisbard. 1989. Appropriate confusion over "brain death." *Journal of the American Medical Association* 261: 2246.

Young, P. J., and B. F. Matta. 2000. Anaesthesia for organ donation in the brainstem dead—why bother? *Anaesthesia* 55: 105–106.

Youngner, S. J., and E. T. Bartlett. 1983. Human death and high technology: The failure of the whole-brain formulations. *Annals of Internal Medicine* 99: 252–258.

Youngner, S. J., C. S. Landefeld, et al. 1989. "Brain death" and organ retrieval. A cross-sectional survey of knowledge and concepts among health professionals. *Journal of the American Medical Association* 261: 2205–2210.

Ysebaert, D., G. V. Beeumen, K. De Greef, et al. 2009. Organ procurement after euthanasia: Belgian experience. *Transplantation Proceedings* 41: 585–586.

Zussman, R. 1992. *Intensive Care: Medical Ethics and the Medical Profession.* Chicago: University of Chicago Press.

Page numbers followed by "*t*" indicates tables.

Printed in the USA/Agawam, MA
January 8, 2013

571731.164